CW01521255

FORTY FIVE IN THE SUN

Forty Five Years of
Medical Practice in a
Tropical Country

Dr Martin Sampath

MINERVA PRESS
MONTREUX   LONDON   WASHINGTON

FORTY FIVE IN THE SUN
Copyright © Dr Martin Sampath 1997

All Rights Reserved

No part of this book may be reproduced in any form
by photocopying or by any electronic or mechanical means,
including information storage or retrieval systems,
without permission in writing from both the copyright
owner and the publisher of this book.

ISBN 1 85863 947 6

First published 1997 by
MINERVA PRESS
195 Knightsbridge
London SW7 1RE

Printed in Great Britain by
Antony Rowe Ltd, Chippenham, Wiltshire

FORTY FIVE IN THE SUN

A Celsius clinical thermometer will placidly register 41 or 42 degrees but will, in Trinidad and Tobago, explode and reveal its mercurial contents at 45 in the sun!

Acknowledgements

I wish to thank my spouse Cynthia for her help, especially after reading the first draft of the manuscript, and my friend and colleague Dr Roderick Thomson for his valuable historical and grammatical corrections of the later version.

Except where specifically indicated, the photographs are the results of my own amateurish efforts – some by delayed action. I am grateful to those who have supplied pictures. Special thanks are due to Mr Shantakumar Takoorcharan of Kumar's Studios, Penal, Trinidad, who has skilfully retrieved recognisable images from fungoid negatives and jaundiced prints nearly half a century old, and for his expert processing of the colour photographs of more recent vintage.

My receptionists, Dharma and Latchmee Naipaul and Aklima Mohammed, have assisted me with information regarding the 'Jharray' ritual, and with the Hindi names of family relationships, and I am indebted to them for this and for their moral support during the preparation of this book.

Lastly, my most profound gratitude is extended to those patients whose forty-five years in the unforgiving sun of our country have unwittingly provided the substance for this work, and to those among them who have so kindly consented to the use of their names and/or photographs.

Martin Sampath
Siparia, Trinidad and Tobago
February 1995

Contents

Prologue	xi
From Yorkshire to Trinidad	13
The Port of Spain Colonial Hospital	18
San Fernando	24
From Delirium to Career Diplomat	37
My Adventures as a District Medical Officer	39
The Civil Service Doctor	43
Private Medical Practice	49
London Interlude	52
Back to General Practice	54
Evidence in Court	57
Foreign Bodies	63
Itching and Scratching	65
Human Wetlands	69
Pox, Malaria, Yellow Fever, Rabies	71
Doctors' Fees	75
A National Health Plan	81
By Any Other Name	85
Shy Patients and Children	87
Anatomical Concepts	90

The Influenzas 94

Cremations 100

Smoking 102

Race Relations 106

Private Practitioners' Advisory Committee 108

AIDS and Sexual Transmission 110

Homosexuals 115

Family Relationships 117

My Prostitute Patients 119

Scorpion Stings and Snake Bites 123

The 'Jharray' Ritual 125

The Trinidad and Tobago Medical Association 128

Ethical, Sociological and Political Aspects of the
      1971-72 Poliomyelitis Epidemic in Trinidad 135

Welcome to Tobago, Doctors! 141

Impotence 146

'Tropical Oils' and Cholesterol 149

A Doctor and His Car 151

The Role of the GP in Providing Primary Care 154

Health and the Trinidad and Tobago Economy 162

When Patients Who Need Transfusion Refuse Blood 168

Medical Examination for Driver's Permit 170

What Constitutes Incapacity to Do One's Work? 173

TTMA Considers The Mount Hope Site
      Unsuitable for a University Complex 181

The Doctor in Politics 185

Women's Travails and Triumphs 191

Is Nuclear Energy Worthwhile? 196

Trinidad and Tobago Medical Association Inaugural
and Honours Dinner at Soong's Great Wall Restaurant
on Sunday, 15th January, 1989 199

Trinidad and Tobago Medical Association: Installation
and Honours Function at the Hilton Hotel on
February 11th, 1984 202

Trinidad and Tobago Medical Association Honours
Ceremony Held at the Hilton Hotel on 7th May, 1988 205

Oration for Dr Percival Harnarayan 207

Oration for Dr Roma Joseph 211

The Dangerous Drugs Bill 216

Crime and Cocaine 229

The Abuse of Children 233

Epilogue 237

Prologue

There are hundreds of doctors in Trinidad and Tobago, better writers than me, with more interesting experiences than mine, who could have written a book such as this. As far as I can discover, two have done so: Drs Crichlow and Tothill, both of San Fernando in the early 1900s. Why only two? Some of those with good intentions may have procrastinated until their spirit became less willing, or their bodies too weak, or a combination of both. Others, with too busy practices, may have died too young and in harness too constricting for reminiscence. I have had the good fortune of having my workload considerably lightened by my competing colleagues in Siparia, Trinidad, before my spirit and body have irretrievably declined, so that I happily now possess the time, the inclination and the energy to set down on paper the remembrances of nearly fifty years.

Like so many of my colleagues, in my time I have played many parts: some of my political and cultural (agricultural and wildlife) experiences have been serially published, and a record of my political involvement is being prepared for publication in book form. (Romantic episodes – such as they have been – remain more or less securely locked up, I hope, in that limbo between the conscious and the subconscious). Yet, these three aspects of my life have inevitably insinuated themselves into some of these medical memories, for compartmentalisation of anyone's life is but an arbitrary convenience, much like the disciplines of medicine itself.

This book is not intended to educate – it is certainly not a General Practitioners' Handbook – its intention is to entertain, even to amuse. Any insight which the reader may gain into the nature of medical practice, or into the psyche of this practitioner during the second half of the twentieth century, in rural Trinidad and Tobago must be regarded as an added bonus.

From Yorkshire to Trinidad

The Cunard luxury liner *Queen Mary*, now a World War II troopship, lay at anchor in Halifax harbour, Nova Scotia, from the eleventh to the sixteenth of September 1944, her enormous length bisected by a church on the foreshore. She had transported Prime Minister Winston Churchill to Canada for an urgent conference with President Franklin D. Roosevelt. Russian and Allied troops were fast approaching Berlin from the East and the West respectively, and these two world leaders had to make important political decisions. Should General Eisenhower be ordered to take Berlin before the Russians got there, or should he be told that Germany's capital city was no longer a military objective and that he should advance dichotomously along the English Channel, knock out the V-weapon bases, occupy the Ruhr, and driving to the East, control the Saar Basin. The disagreements between Montgomery and Eisenhower over military strategy, also required delicate diplomacy at the highest political level. At this second Quebec conference, code named 'Octagon'[1], they were to be the guests of Canadian Prime Minister Mr McKenzie King.

Not far away from the *Queen Mary*, a tiny Elders and Fyfe line banana boat named the *Tilapia* (after a species of Malayan fish), was moored to the quay, and laden with bacon in her cold storage compartments instead of the luxury tropical fruit. On board were four West Indian medical students and two young English ladies, who had been evacuated as children when invasion by Hitler seemed imminent, an invalid lady, accompanied by her nurse, and a few others, making a total of twelve passengers all bound for Britain.

We four students had completed two years' pre-medical studies at McGill University in Montreal, and had been awarded Colonial

---

[1] The partition of Germany, and the consideration of the Morgenthau proposal for the ruralisation of that country, were also on the 'Octagon' agenda.

Development and Welfare scholarships, tenable at British medical schools. We had signed an agreement to return to the West Indies after graduation to practise our profession in our homeland for five years. Marjorie Johnson, Rodney Mahabir and I were from Trinidad, and Tony Gale was from Barbados.

We remained aboard the cramped vessel, against the jetty, under strict security, for two days and nights awaiting sailing orders, for it was believed that Halifax was swarming with Nazi spies. Suddenly and unexpectedly, for the wind was rising and the moored ship was rocking and knocking uncomfortably against the planks of the dock, we headed out to sea with huge waves breaking over our bow. We pushed out of the harbour into the North Atlantic where a violent storm was raging.

Three months before, in just such a storm on D-Day, the allied invasion fleets had crossed the Channel, taking Hitler and his generals by complete surprise. Like many of the members of the invasion, we passengers were violently seasick and emerged on deck, only after four days, to enjoy the fresh air, the grey but beautiful ocean, and the majestic sight of seventy-four other ships around us. We were in a convoy escorted by two aircraft carriers – converted grain ships – each carrying a couple of Swordfish spotter planes armed with rockets and machine guns. In the event, we encountered no submarines. The medical students were entertained – presumably because of our status as potential professionals – at the Captain's table, where we had much interesting discourse with the youthful First Mate.

We landed at Liverpool, after a fortnight's sailing, then continued to London by train. London: permanent nightly blackouts, shells of bombed out and burnt-out buildings everywhere, with open water tanks wherever there was a space. London, after the blitz and the 'Doodlebugs', as the V-1s were contemptuously named by the heroic Londoners. We arrived at almost the same time as the V-2s, the progenitors of modern day space rockets and intercontinental ballistic missiles. We attended the hundredth showing of *Arsenic and Old Lace* – no player being a member of the original cast. In a London restaurant, we discovered that 'Vienna Steak' was fried hamburger, and the 'Stewed Fruit' of the menu was rhubarb.

Marjorie Johnson and Tony Gale were posted to Birmingham; Rodney Mahabir and I went to Leeds.

I shall always treasure the memory of my five and a half years in Leeds and its environs, the warmth and camaraderie of my fellow students, and the hospitality of their parents and of the general public. The people of Yorkshire are truly the salt of the earth.

I graduated MB, Ch.B. in March 1950 and immediately received by post, from the Colonial Office in London, my steamship ticket to Trinidad and an official order to report to the Director of Medical Services in Port of Spain. I began my round of goodbyes to my many friends and favourite professors and lecturers. One of these, a New Zealander, Archibald Durward, Professor of Anatomy, I located in the dissecting room in the process of conducting a *viva voce* examination of half a dozen students, all sitting on the customary high stools around a partly dissected subject. The prof was famous for his blunt and ready wit. He once told us the story of a Maori anatomy professor colleague of his who during an address told his audience: "You may think that I am a full-blooded Maori – but I am not: I have Scottish blood in me: my grandfather once ate a missionary!"

As I shook Professor Durward's hand, he said to me, "So now you are licensed to kill as well as cure?"

"Yes sir," I replied, and looking at the corpse I added, "And to do post mortems!"

"Touché!" he exclaimed and exploded into laughter, his students around the dissecting table joining in with gusto, much to the consternation of the examiners and students at the other tables in the large dissecting room, which traditionally was a grave and silent place.

World War II was long over and the Cold War was at its height. Mao Tse-Tung was master of mainland China, and trouble was brewing in Korea, but all was quiet on the English front. So that when I boarded my ship at Southampton[2], in April 1950, in marked contrast with wartime Halifax in 1944, not only were the date and time of departure published well in advance, but also the passenger list and the cabins to which the travellers had been assigned.

---

[2] It was from Southampton, and nearby Portsmouth, that British and United States troops sailed to meet the rest of the invasion fleet at 'Area Z' in the English Channel – also known as 'Piccadilly Circus' – for Operation 'Neptune', the assault on Normandy.

If this had been a work of fiction, the string of coincidences which I am about to relate would have assured its summary rejection by any self-respecting publisher: the ship was SS *Matina*, a banana boat of the Elders and Fyfe line. Two young doctors were allocated the Governor's Stateroom. I was one and the other – have you guessed? – Dr Tony Gale of Barbados and Birmingham, whom I had not seen for five and a half years. We were, as in 1944, seated at the table headed by the Captain, with whom we later had much interesting discourse. And who was the Captain of the *Matina*? Well, he turned out to be the former First Mate of the good old SS *Tilapia!*

After a pleasantly uneventful fortnight, we approached the island of Barbados, but we were not to call there, and as we sailed past, Tony Gale stared wistfully at the island he hadn't seen for over seven years. On our starboard side, the clear blue waters were breaking tantalisingly into foam on Barbados's coral sands. Tony asked me about Trinidad and whether we had beaches such as those. I replied that on our north and north-east coasts, our beaches were almost as lovely as his, but the others, around the island, were usually muddied by our own rivers and by the Orinoco of Venezuela which was, at one point, a mere seven miles away.

Early the next morning, we could see the Northern Range of Trinidad, and within the hour, the *Matina* left the clear waters of the Caribbean Sea, manoeuvred the narrow passage of the Small Boca (Spanish for 'mouth'), and entered the Gulf of Paria. Soon, our propeller was churning up the mud of Port of Spain harbour, and we were presently alongside the dock.

When I was a boy, there was no deep water harbour. The ships rode at anchor several miles out and were approached by cargo and passengers in lighters and motor launches. The story is told about a debate in our Legislative Council, when a government member told the legislators that a channel would be dredged deep enough to enable large vessels coming in from the Gulf to moor alongside the jetty. A certain member, elected more for his local popularity as a wrestler than for his erudition, enquired how this channel would be marked so that ships should not run aground. On being told that the authority would arrange for buoys with lanterns at night, the enquiring member was outraged.

"For such an important job," he asked, "wouldn't it be better to have grown men instead?"

Looking down from the deck of the Matina, we could see hundreds of men, women and children of all shades of complexion and styles of attire: Kurtahs, dhotis and three-piece suits stood side by side. There was singing of hymns and waving of palm leaves. Whom were they expecting? Surely there was no Jesus Christ or other Messiah on board? I then remembered that one of our group, an Afro-Trinidadian, had been visited at Southampton by British Secret Servicemen (as we were told), and his luggage and cabin thoroughly searched. The reception on the dock was for a famous politician – a dedicated opponent of Colonial rule, named Tubal Uriah Buzz Butler, who had been unsuccessfully tried for treason in Trinidad and who, at that time, was in exile in Britain. He was expected to return on that day, but had instead sent one of his lieutenants. As fate would have it, Butler and I were opposing candidates for election to the Federal Parliament of the West Indies some seventeen years later.

I searched with my eyes among the teeming crowd, and there was *my* reception committee in a tight bunch: my father, mother, Uncle Shadrack (a medical doctor), my Aunt Celestina (an optician) and my three sisters, all grown up. The youngest, Christabelle, who had been the shortest of the three when I left home, was now the tallest. Among them was a little boy whom I guessed to be my youngest brother, Ronald, born when I was in Canada.

I had visions of spending at least a week with my family, going with them to some of our beaches, catching up with domestic happenings and national events, soaking up some sunshine, and leaching away, with clean fresh air, some of the smog of Leeds and London from my lungs. This was not to be. The very next day a telegram signed by Dr A. A. Peat, Director of Medical Services, arrived, ordering me to report at once to his office. On arrival, I was informed that I was to take up duties as a Grade 'C' officer at the Colonial Hospital, Port of Spain, forty miles away from my home town, San Fernando.

"What about the San Fernando Hospital?" I asked. "It would be much more convenient for me!"

It would have to be Port of Spain, I was told: their need was greater than mine.

The Port of Spain Colonial Hospital

Before relating some of my experiences at this hospital, it would be useful to outline very briefly the general set up of institutions and other agencies involved in medical care in the Crown Colony of Trinidad and Tobago, and their relationship with other colonial agencies in the year 1950.

The Department of Health was one of the many government departments in existence as part of the Civil Service. There were, for example, departments of Agriculture, Public Works and Hydraulics, Education and so on, each with a Director and one or more Deputy Directors. The co-ordinating agency was the Colonial Secretary's Office, the Col. Sec. himself being next in command to the Governor, and indeed often acting as Governor during that official's absence from the Colony. To become the Colonial Secretary was the final hurdle in the journey to the top post, and many of our Col. Secs. were posted as Governors to other of His Majesty's colonies.

In 1950, the Directors and Deputies of these departments were invariably white or near white. The health departments were striking exceptions to this race/colour convention: the Director, Dr Peat, was a brown skinned, negro-white mixture, from Jamaica. One Deputy, in charge of Public Health, Dr Sankerali, was an Indo-Trinidadian, and the other Deputy, Dr Waterman, in charge of curative medicine, was also brown skinned with a touch perhaps of non-white ancestry. Both of these deputies were eminent practitioners in their respective fields: Dr Sankerali in Public Health and Sanitation, and Dr Waterman in Obstetrics and Gynaecology. They had each, in turn, acted as Director, and Dr Sankerali had actually been permanently appointed to that post, but unfortunately died before he could take up the appointment.

When I joined the service, I must confess that my ambition as a non-white colonial was, after my stint in clinical medicine, to take a diploma in Public Health and eventually become Director of Medical Services. No non-white colonial could aspire to anything higher without having his sanity questioned!

The Medical Services were widespread: on the clinical side there were three large colonial hospitals situated in Port of Spain, San Fernando and Scarborough, Tobago. There were several smaller district hospitals and health offices, all over the two islands, run by 'District Medical Officers' (DMOs). At the colonial hospitals, the doctors were classified into three grades: the Grade 'A' physicians and surgeons were the consultants and were allowed to carry on private practices. In addition to their hospital work, their private practice was done very informally and largely at the hospitals during regular Government hours. The Grade 'B' Medicos had postgraduate qualifications, and were on their way to the higher grade, but until then, they were not allowed private practice and private fees. The Grade 'C' doctors were the newcomers who did all the donkey work, put in the longest hours for the lowest pay, but learned more medicine and did more surgery in a month than they had during their entire sojourn at medical school. The DMOs were allowed unlimited private practice, received their monthly civil service salaries, and had other perks and emoluments which I shall describe later. It was the immediate ambition of most Grade 'C's to act in the district for a few months, save a little money, then decide whether to stay in the Service towards a Grade 'A' appointment, seek a permanent DMO appointment, or go fully into private practice. The conditions of work at the hospitals were so unattractive that only a small percentage of recruits stayed on.

On the Public Health side, there was approximately one Medical Officer of Health (MOH) for each county and each municipality, and this doctor was in charge of all aspects of sanitation, inoculations and other preventive measures in his district. He was not allowed to do private practice.

There were two Grade 'C' doctors at the Port of Spain hospital when I took up duties there: these were Dr Arneaud, whom I knew from St Mary's College, Trinidad, and McGill, Canada, and Dr Simon Ramesar, who was my friend from Trinidad, McGill, and who, while at Sheffield in England, had visited me in Leeds. He had married a Canadian girl and she had accompanied him to England and back to Trinidad. He and his family lived in the hospital compound and they were extremely helpful to me in many ways during those rigorous, and often lonely, days in Port of Spain.

We were each put in charge of two in-patient wards under the direct supervision of the appropriate consultant. My boss was Dr Aldwyn G. Francis, a Grade 'A' officer who inspected my notes on the patients' record sheets, checked my diagnoses and prescriptions, and wrote his comments and corrections for my edification and the patients' safety! I shall always be grateful to him for his diplomatic and erudite guidance.

Our duties included a twenty-four hour stint in the casualty department, followed by an eight-hour session as anaesthetist in the operating theatre. 'Casualty' was, to put it mildly, something of a misnomer: apart from accident cases legitimately entering there – from bruised elbows to multiple compound fractures and stab wounds – everything from common colds to typhoid fever applied to that department for medical attention, with and without referrals. In 1950, there was only one doctor in casualty at any one time. Grade 'C' officers did this twice per week; the other nights were serviced by part-time private doctors, some of them recent graduates who had served a year or so at the hospital, and had gone out into private practice, and others who had passed the retirement age, but could not bear to stay away from their profession. I was privileged to meet one of the latter, as he came in at four in the afternoon to take over from me. He was Dr Jesse Grell, an Englishman who had been the DMO for Siparia when I was an infant. He had vaccinated me – among thousands of other babies in that district – against smallpox. When I showed him the three scars on my left upper arm, this kind old Britisher spontaneously held me to his chest in an emotional hug. Only now, when I meet grown men and women whom I myself vaccinated or delivered forty years ago, do I understand the emotions which must have assailed this kind old man that day in the casualty department.

All medical services, including drugs and operations at Government institutions, were absolutely free of cost. The volume and stress in the casualty department were, therefore, easy to understand. There were two exceptions to the no-charge policy: a small fee was levied for the use of the private rooms at the hospitals.

There existed a parallel system of doctors and nursing homes in many parts of the islands, but the volume of clients handled at these places was minuscule compared with the hospitals and health offices. At these last offices, an 'assessment' of each patient was made by the clerk in attendance, and, at his sole discretion, a charge of one shilling was levied on some of them.

How we, young, inexperienced newcomers, survived and maintained our sanity amid the tense and often chaotic conditions in casualty, has always been a source of wonderment to me. I am sure that some of us must have developed an immunity – a callousness approaching schizophrenia – after our stint in that place.

The second half of the twenty-four hour shift from about nine in the evening to eight in the morning, was usually relatively quiet. During this period, proper emergencies would come in – both medical and surgical. As the casualty officer was the only doctor on duty in the entire hospital, emergencies in the wards were also his responsibility. The consultants were on call on a rota basis, and in our inexperience, we often got the Surgeon-on-Duty out of bed quite unnecessarily. He was appropriately called the SOD.

One morning, at about two o'clock, the ward sister called me to see an aborting woman who was bleeding profusely. She had already set up a glucose-saline drip on her own initiative – a procedure usually frowned upon in England – and then talked me through my first placenta removal and uterine curettage. She also handed me the ergometrine laden syringe for injection. During my stay at the hospitals, I was always impressed by the high standard of the nurses – both local and foreign; were it not for them, medical attention at the hospitals would surely have collapsed long before 1950.

I boarded at a guest house on the same street as the hospital, and a ten minute walk away. It was run by a matronly Miss Stollmeyer. I had a small room, just large enough to accommodate a narrow bed, a small desk and a tiny clothes closet. This, and three substantial, nutritious meals per day, cost $100 per month. My monthly salary was to be $280, before tax.

The people I used to know in Port of Spain, when I left for Canada in 1942, had all gone elsewhere or were inaccessible, for one reason or another, and my social life was non-existent. I discovered that a friend of mine was working at the same hospital, as a nutritionist. I knew her as a member of my literary club called the Minerva Club, in the city, whom I met several times in Montreal up until 1944, and whom I liked very much. She was the girlfriend of a close friend of mine, and so I never had any romantic association with her. I invited her up to my small room, as she appeared to be unattached – my friend had married someone else. This young lady was quite attractive and excellent company. We sat, on the narrow bed, and chatted about old times in Trinidad and Canada, and I put my arms around her, hoping that close physical contact – added to the mental rapport we had already established – would elevate both my mood and my libido. Alas, all it did was to remind me of Leeds and my friends there. I was thoroughly and depressingly homesick for Yorkshire !

Among the guests at Miss Stollmeyer's were three lovely Venezuelan girls employed at their country's embassy in the city. One of them owned a Hillman Minx motor car and they invited me to accompany them to the Perseverance Club in the beautiful Diego Martin Valley, a verdant suburb three miles out of Port of Spain. This club had a standing orchestra and a dance floor. We visited this enchanted setting twice per week – the ladies were expert dancers and flawlessly followed every movement, from tango to Viennese waltz, and it was this activity which gradually curbed my debilitating yearning for the North Riding and its wonderful human beings.

My first experience of civil service apathy and inefficiency came at the end of the month. The pay clerk came around with the doctors' envelopes and there was none for me! My landlady was expecting her $100, and I was almost broke. On enquiring from the Lay Secretary of the hospital, I was told nonchalantly that such delay was not unusual; my appointment was being processed and my money was safe. I would receive two or three month's salary all at once. I was incensed: as far as I was concerned, I was hounded down to start work as soon as I arrived, everyone knew that I was coming and when I was doing so. If the service of doctors was so urgently required, could not the Director of Medical Services be interested enough in the welfare of his recruits to ensure that their appointments were processed in time for the payment of their first salaries?

I told the Lay Secretary that if I was not paid that same afternoon – it was about two o'clock – I would leave the hospital immediately at four o'clock and never return. He could see from the expression on my face that I meant every word I said, that this was no idle threat. He made two phone calls and took me in his car to the Treasury building which was five minutes away. There he spoke to two of the officials and sat with me, exchanging pleasantries about my acclimatisation to the Trinidad weather. After half an hour, one of the tellers nodded to him and he said to me, "Doctor, your appointment has been finalised. The teller in that cage is ready for you."

San Fernando

After three months in Port of Spain, my request for a transfer to my home town, San Fernando, was granted. The casualty department there was even more chaotic than in the big city hospital. Patients were rushing in on the doctor from all sides, some virtually brandishing their referrals in the poor medico's face. Queuing was apparently unheard of, and the ward sister and wardsmen were helpless against the noisy assault. There were three other casualty officers: Drs Harry Seenath, Herbert Barrow and Mavis Rampersad. We thoroughly reorganised the casualty department by isolating the waiting room, having the nurse give out numbers to the patients upon their arrival, and allowing only one entrance to the examination room. Within a month, things were like clockwork. The atmosphere at the southern hospital was strikingly different from that in the north: the camaraderie between senior doctors, their juniors, nursing staff, lay staff and even wardsmen was excellent. Each one eagerly gave the other a helping hand beyond what would normally be expected of his or her station.

The Grade 'C' officers were given free rein to run the casualty department and we prepared our own monthly rotas. It was a pleasure to work in such an environment, and living at home with my parents and siblings made life seem to me to be the fulfilment of all I could desire. The hours were long, and the salary was meagre, but I was a bachelor with very few commitments and many friends. We arranged our rota so that each of us would have a long weekend off every month – our duties at the hospital were performed in our absence by a designated colleague. My boss, consultant physician Dr George Wattley, was energetic, competent, conscientious, kind and considerate. His contribution to my further medical education and his example in dedication and efficiency I shall always treasure.

My long weekends were usually spent with my family at my uncle Dr Shadrack's beach house on the east coast, at Mayaro. The other doctors spent theirs similarly, at their own venues. Tragedy struck, however, when our fellow doctor, Herbert Barrow, drowned at Toco, on the north-east tip of the island, during his weekend off. Apparently, he collapsed just as he succeeded in getting his drowning daughter safely into the shallows. His distraught widow said to me, "And I thought it was such a good thing that you were holding on for him." When I first heard the sad news I went quietly alone into the doctors' common room and wept: such was the relationship we fostered at San Fernando.

I mentioned earlier that Grade 'A' doctors were allowed to do private work at the hospitals. Not long before his death, Dr Barrow was sitting with us in the common room, at about ten in the morning, sipping the customary grapefruit juice prepared for us as a mid-morning refreshment. We often took off our long white coats for this ritual. Herbert, having finished his drink, got up, retrieved a coat from among the others on the rack, and went out. Within two minutes, he rushed in again, hurriedly took off his coat and, replacing it on the rack, put on another. We were all greatly puzzled by this, and asked him to explain. "Boy!" said he, "When I put my hand into the pocket I pulled out masses of five dollar notes!" He had inadvertently donned the coat of Sir Henry Pierre, eminent consultant surgeon whose coat happened to be about the same size as his.

Dr Pierre's fame as a surgeon had spread throughout the Caribbean. During the United States sojourn in Trinidad for World War II, he did surgery for their troops on many occasions and was officially honoured by them on their departure from their Army and Navy bases. He was knighted by King George VI for his outstanding contribution to surgery. He never lost the common touch and was extremely popular with his colleagues and his patients alike. He did not actively seek payments from his patients – the numerous five dollar bills he received were more often than not regarded by his clients as gifts rather than fees.

Because of the prevailing culture – as a result, perhaps, of the conditions of slavery and indenture, especially the latter – there was little distinction in the minds of the more plebeian of our population between fees, gifts and bribes. A few years ago, one of my friends and political colleagues, now an elected member of parliament, and a former Minister of Government, told me that when he was a boy of about twelve years of age, he was under my care at the San Fernando hospital suffering from typhoid fever. He had been referred to the hospital by my general practitioner uncle, Dr Shadrack Sampath. The boy's father brought me a substantial gift of poultry and eggs, and asked me to give the lad the best treatment available. I had refused the gift, telling the father that his son would get the best treatment regardless, and that the food should be used for his family whom I felt needed it more than I did. The father was hurt – perhaps I had unwittingly insulted him by not accepting his kind gift. I had no recollection at all of this incident, but I know that I never accepted gifts from patients, either of goods or of money. My friend completed his story by telling me that his father took the gifts to my uncle with the same request, and my uncle, wiser than me in the psychology and sociology of the population, accepted the gift. Knowing my uncle, I am sure that he must have quickly found some deserving family by whom the food would be gratefully accepted.

Sir Henry Pierre's teacher and mentor was Dr Peter Rostant, a white French Creole veteran of World War I. He had been at the hospital for many decades and upon his retirement had written an unpublished history of that institution. In 1950, he carried on his private general practice in San Fernando, and worked part-time in paediatric surgery at the hospital. I occasionally enjoyed the privilege of giving the anaesthetic while Drs Pierre and Rostant, both eminent men, student and former teacher, black and white respectively, worked together in the operating theatre. Dr Rostant often acted as superintendent of the hospital during his former student's absence. He had a fine sense of humour: a plate on the back of his car read, 'If you can read this you are too damn close'.

At a time when white domination was the mode accepted by whites, blacks and browns alike, and equality of opportunity was the dream only of radicals, Dr Peter Rostant was an active and persistent proponent of fair and equal treatment for all with whom he came into contact: he was responsible for the admission to employment of several non-white doctors, for example, in jobs with salaries that at that time were normally reserved for white expatriates in large oil companies.

The Grade 'C' salary of $280 per month, we found to be too low, especially in view of the overtime, night and weekend duties. Our emoluments compared very unfavourably with corresponding members of the civil service, who worked from nine until four, sometimes half-days on Saturdays, and never on Sundays or public holidays. We wrote repeatedly to the Director of Medical Services asking that we should be paid extra for the comparative extra hours we put in. The following correspondence, which arose out of an incident in which I was involved, reflects our predicament, our frustrations and importantly, our solidarity:

From: *Supt. Medical Officer (Specialist),*
             Col. Hosp., San Fernando

To: *Dr M.S. Sampath, Col. Hosp., San Fernando*

Dated: *27 December, 1951*

Subject: *Refusal of Police Surgeon and Casualty Officer,*
             Colonial Hospital, San Fernando,
             to examine drunken driver

1. *With reference to correspondence of the above subject ending with your minute dated 12th December, 1951, I am directed by the Director of Medical Services to inform you that he does not at all subscribe to the cavalier fashion in which this case was handled by you, and that it is the duty of every public officer to see to it that Government medical work, particularly those involving breaches of the laws of the country, are properly and efficiently executed.*

2. *In his view the question as to whether it was your particular duty to do the work or not, does not obviate your taking an intelligent interest in the proceedings. Moreover, he wishes it to be clearly understood that whenever the Police Surgeon is absent or is unable to do the particular duty, it is clearly in the interest of efficiency that any Government Officer consulted should assist.*

3. *He thinks that in courtesy, you should have spoken direct to Dr Mejias before neglecting to do the work, and sending the*

man out on the street to be dealt with in whatever manner the police pleased.

(Signed)
H.C. Shepherd
Supt. Medical Officer (Specialist)

*

Colonial Hospital, San Fernando
January 12, 1952

The Director of Medical Services
Through: S.M.O.(S), San Fernando

Sir,

RE: REFUSAL OF POLICE SURGEON AND CASUALTY
         OFFICER TO EXAMINE DRUNKEN DRIVER

I beg to refer to your communication of December 27th 1951, to make the following observations and to ask the following questions:

1. *With reference to your statement, 'I do not at all subscribe to the cavalier fashion in which this case was handled by you'.*

   I am deeply hurt by your choice of words. I was on duty from 8.30 a.m. that day, and had been attending to a steady stream of patients, many of them requiring considerable effort and concentration.

   On that Saturday, at 8.50 p.m., when the man Outridge was brought into the Casualty Department, there were, awaiting attention several sick and injured persons, some of them critically ill. I submit a list of the cases seen by me and the times when examination and treatment were completed. You will observe that it was 1.50 a.m., Sunday, before I was able to sit down and take a rest from my immediate labours.

Name	Diagnosis, treatment & disposal	Time
Bhagmaniya	Incised wound of forearm with cut tendons. Sutured and discharged	8.15 p.m.
Outridge	Request by police for examination for drunkenness: Referred to Police Surgeon	8.50 p.m.
McKeckie	Ruptured appendix – admitted to Ward 5	9.05 p.m.
Sammy	Cutlass wounds on eyebrow and thumb. Sutured and discharged	9.15 p.m.
Guevara	Incised and lacerated wounds on lip. Sutured and discharged	9.40 p.m.
Phelps	Acute tonsillitis: treated and discharged	9.45 p.m.
Moore	Pneumonia: admitted to Ward 8	9.50 p.m.
Robain	Splinter in thumb. Removed, sutured and discharged	10.10 p.m.
Drakes	Lacerations of hand involving tendons, lacerations of shoulder and head. Sutured and discharged	11.30 p.m.
Barrat	Haematoma of eyelids and eyeballs. Treated and discharged	11.40 p.m.
Hughes	Lacerations of forehead. Sutured and discharged	11.40 p.m.
Jusuip	Strangulated hernia. Reduction attempted, admitted to Ward 11	12.00 mn
Young	Cut throat, involving large veins and severing sterno-mastoid. Shock treated, sutured in Casualty, admitted to Ward 5	1.10 a.m.
Joseph	Hysterical unconsciousness. Treated and discharged	1.20 a.m.
Sukhdeo	Laceration and haematoma of forehead. Sutured and discharged	1.40 a.m.
de Lande	Scorpion sting. Treated and discharged	1.50 a.m.

In addition, I attended and treated several emergencies in the wards. I have no record of these and am therefore unable to add them to this list.

In my original comment to you on this matter, I made a general statement to the above effect: I felt that, in the event of your deciding that I was guilty of the slightest neglect of duty in refusing to examine Outridge, you should have asked me to describe in greater detail the circumstances of the incident, before making such a harsh, and I feel unfair criticism of my conduct and casting such a slur on my character. I feel, therefore, that I must ask you to reconsider your opinion.

2. *'...it is the duty of every public officer to see to it that Government medical work, particularly those involving breaches of the laws of the country, are properly and efficiently executed.'*

   I appreciate the importance and I entirely agree with the sentiment of this statement. I submit, however, that the responsibility for specific duties must rest with officers specifically detailed to do these duties, and that they cannot be left in the nebulous phase of all Government officers seeing to it that all the work is efficiently executed. If one should carry the general concept to its logical conclusion, one should accept with equanimity the situation which would arise when any DMO neglects or refuses to do his own work and on the slightest pretext, sends his patients to a hospital.

   Indeed, such an unqualified principle can be abused to the point where no DMO needs to do any public work at all, so long as patients can find their way, or be escorted to a hospital.

3. *'The question as to whether it was your particular duty to do the work or not does not obviate your taking an intelligent interest in the proceedings'.*

   I have taken the liberty of interpreting this to mean, 'Although it was not your duty to do the work, you should have taken an intelligent interest in the proceedings'.

*With reference to the second part of the statement, please
permit me again to call your attention to the foregoing list.
You will observe that it would have been several hours before I
could have been justified in dealing with the strictly medico-
legal matter of examining an alleged drunken driver – albeit an
examination lasting only ten to fifteen minutes. I trust you
would not hold that assisting in building up a case for the
police in an incident involving a traffic offence was more urgent
and important than the immediate tasks before me, of
preserving life and limb. You will agree that this is precisely
why the post of Police Surgeon exists in all civilised countries
as distinct from, and not encroaching on that of, Casualty
Officer.*

*You have yourself stated in a press release that for Casualty
Officers, night duties are extra duties: are we also to take on
the duties of Police Surgeon during the night ?*

*I hope it will not appear presumptuous for me to suggest that,
in the present instance, I exhibited a certain intelligent interest,
when I did the only thing which would benefit both my ill
patients and the police viz.: to send the driver immediately back
to the Police Surgeon before he could recover from his alleged
alcoholic state.*

*The crux of the matter is surely this: Dr Mejias refused to
examine the man because this man was a friend of his. Do you
rule that he was therefore **unable** to do the particular duty?*

4. *'You should have spoken direct to Dr Mejias before neglecting
   to do the work and sending the man out on the street to be dealt
   with in whatever manner the police pleased'.*

*I agree that it would have been more polite for me to have
spoken direct to Dr Mejias. However, I trust you will
understand why, under the pressure of such circumstances as I
have described, I found it difficult to exhibit a courtesy which
was entirely ignored by this senior officer.*

Yet it is incumbent upon me to deny that the man was sent out on the street to be dealt with in whatever manner the police pleased. I told the policeman that it was not part of my duties to do this work and that the man should be taken back to the police surgeon.

I must also point out that the police were doing whatever they pleased with the man, from the time they apprehended him, and my advice as to how he should be treated, was never sought; I therefore resent the implication that I was, at any time, responsible for any part of the police behaviour towards the man.

*Surely, the onus was on the Police Surgeon to make arrangements for the examination of any person referred to him by the police, and in cases where, for any reason, he felt he could not do **his own work**, to write, phone or call personally on some other officer, and solicit his assistance.*

Please allow me to suggest that this incident makes it clear that if the duties of Police Surgeons, district medical officers and hospital officers, are not precisely defined, and without ambiguity, all Government medical work will become everybody's business and nobody's particular responsibility, and that the efficiency of the medical services will further deteriorate.

In the interest of the medical services, and of my own reputation, I ask, therefore, that you give an early ruling on the following points:-

(a) *Was Dr Mejias justified in refusing to examine Outridge?*

(b) *Is a DMO permitted to send a case to hospital without a letter or some clear form of reference?*

(c) *Is it the duty of the Casualty Officer to examine persons brought to him by the police with a request to determine:*

> (i)   Whether the person is under the influence of alcohol?
> or   (ii)   Whether the person has been raped?
> or   (iii)   Whether the person's clothing contains semen or blood?
> or   (iv)   Whether there are marks of violence?

(d)   Is it the duty of the Casualty Officer to examine and treat children, presented by their mothers to him, because it is children's clinic day and there is no doctor at the children's clinic?

(e)   Is it the duty of the Casualty Officer to examine and treat persons presenting themselves to him with the statement that there is no doctor at the Health Office?

(f)   Is it the duty of the Casualty Officer to treat sick policemen who cannot find the Police Surgeon?

(g)   Is it the duty of the Casualty Officer to examine and treat prisoners in custody?

I ask these questions with a note of urgency because I am often called upon to perform these duties and I thank you, in anticipation again for an early reply.

I have the honour to be, Sir
Your obedient servant

(Signed)
Martin S. Sampath

CASUALTY OFFICER

*

I informed my Grade 'C' colleagues about the incident and showed them the above correspondence. They sent the following letter to the Director:

Colonial Hospital, San Fernando
January 12 1952

The Director of Medical Services
Through S.M.O. (S)
San Fernando

RE: REFUSAL OF POLICE SURGEON AND CASUALTY
      OFFICER TO EXAMINE DRUNKEN DRIVER

1. *Following this incident, which has been brought to our attention, we wish to state that, under the circumstances as set out in detail by Dr Sampath, the criticisms of his attitude in the matter are unmerited.*

2. *It has been, throughout our experience in hospital service here, the unfortunate and additional burden of the Casualty Medical Officers to deal with innumerable cases that should ordinarily be dealt with by DMOs, and Police Surgeons, in the course of their duties. We have done that, sometimes with philosophic acceptance, and sometimes with actual protest to the Supt. Medical Officer (Specialist). We find in this case, however, that a Casualty Officer is actually held culpable for not performing the duties of some other Government Medical Officer at a time when that medical officer refused to do his duty on a most frivolous excuse, and at a time when the Casualty Officer was most busily engaged in performing his own urgent duties.*

3. *We feel sure that your attitude to the Casualty Officer can only have arisen as a result of non-appraisal of the true situation, and we feel that Dr Sampath's resentment of the manner in which he has been dealt with is fully justified.*

4. *As the matter now stands, the duties of the Casualty Officer are all embracing – a condition which leads to gross inefficiency and dissatisfaction. We would be pleased if this particular aspect be cleared up, and some definite ruling made which will make the answers to Dr Sampath's questions lucid, and the*

*general procedure of the Casualty Officer one that can be
readily accepted and followed.*

*We have the honour to be, Sir
Your obedient servants,*

*(Signed)
Herbert Barrow
Noble L. Sarkar
P. Harnarayan.*

Our entreaties, including the last, were consistently ignored: we never had the courtesy of an acknowledgement of our letters, far less some sort of investigation or reply. So, in desperation, the south doctors wrote to their northern counterparts outlining a plan which we formulated for withholding our labour during all periods before nine in the morning and after four in the afternoon (Civil Service hours of work), and after twelve noon on Saturdays and all day Sundays and public holidays, unless our request for overtime for work performed outside Civil Service hours was agreed upon. We suggested a date, two months from then, as a deadline for agreement.

Not only did the northern doctors not agree to our plan, they leaked it to the Director! He agreed only to an increase for all Grade 'C' officers to $300 per month, regardless of former service, so that those with four years' service got the same salary as those just joining! This was an obvious ploy to set the seniors against the juniors. In addition, the northern doctors were almost immediately awarded lucrative study leaves for postgraduate qualifications while the protesting southerners were left in the cold!

There was a chronic shortage of doctors at both hospitals, and the workload was almost unbearable. The difference between the earnings of the private practitioner and the government doctor was enormous – an average ratio of six to one! So most civil service doctors were transients in the hospitals, and everyone knew this. It is not surprising, then, that doctors who tried to improve conditions in these institutions were few. After all, the more chaos there was in government institutions, the more would be the demand for private medical attention.

When the reasons for the rapid exodus of medical recruits was pointed out to the Director, his cynical reply was, "Oh, let them leave: when private practice becomes overcrowded, and they start starving, they will be begging to come back to the hospital!"

It has taken forty years for his prediction to come to pass, and it has done so, not so much as a result of the dilution of private practice, but because the rebounding slump following the oil boom, with its unshakeable inflation, has caused unemployment to rise to over 25%, while the cost of living has remained at oil-boom heights. People just do not have the money to consult a private doctor, the health offices and hospitals are grossly overcrowded, and the chaos is as bad, or even worse, than it was in the 1950s.

Despite the strenuous workload, I enjoyed my stay at San Fernando very much. Early in 1952, I was promoted to act as a Grade 'B' officer at the princely salary of $400 per month. When I elatedly told my uncle of my good fortune, he replied, "I know you enjoy your very interesting work at the hospital, but really you ought to know that, on some days, I collect more than that!" He must have had a tremendous practice and I knew that, on some days, he didn't leave his office until eight in the evening. His fees, incidentally, were two dollars per consultation, and three dollars if he had to give an injection. He gave a prescription to be filled at the patient's expense at any nearby pharmacy.

From Delirium to Career Diplomat

Of the many interesting cases which I treated at the hospitals, there is one which I recall with exceptional satisfaction.

A lad of sixteen was brought to the casualty department by his brothers one night, in delirium with a very high fever. I admitted him to my ward and began treatment with Atebrine – the standard treatment for malaria in those days, which was used as a therapeutic test for that disease, that was endemic in 1950s Trinidad. There was no response in the first twelve hours. The young man became comatose, alternating with severe agitation, would swallow nothing, and kept waving his arms about and shouting out quite comprehensible phrases, which suggested that he was having visual hallucinations. He was a brilliant student in the Form Five O-level class at Naparima College, a secondary school adjoining the hospital. His brothers had given me a history which revealed that he had been having these hallucinations at home on the previous day: they were convinced that he was 'going out of his head', as he kept saying, among other things, that a spaceship had landed in their front yard. As he lay in the ward, it was obvious that dehydration, toxicity and exhaustion would end his young life if this condition continued much longer. I called my colleague, Dr Russell Barrow, whose skill in anaesthesiology was well known, and outlined the following plan: the nurses and wardsmen would hold the patient down, Dr Barrow would administer a small intravenous dose of Pentothal, and when he was quiet, a glucose saline drip would be started through the same needle. It worked like a charm, and during the night the nurses were able to give him three litres of the fluid. The following morning, the fever was gone, but his restlessness and hallucinations persisted. We had no psychiatric facilities at the hospital at that time, and in order to get him to the St Ann's Psychiatric Hospital, forty miles away, the law required that he be legally certified as being insane by a magistrate. I contacted Mr J. Brathwaite, magistrate of San Fernando, and later a High Court judge, who agreed to come with me to see the patient. I remember that day as clearly as if it were yesterday: it had been raining non-stop since early morning, and I collected Mr Brathwaite in my little Hillman car P.B.2916. The memory I carry of that trip from the courthouse to the hospital is of the windscreen wipers going at full speed, with my headlights on, and the driving white downpour rattling against the glass. Mr Brathwaite looked at my statement and the patient and signed the authorisation.

After taking the magistrate back to his court, I procured an ambulance and, accompanied by a nurse and the ambulance driver, we took the lad to St Ann's. We were received by Dr Roget de Verteuil, who happened to be a former student colleague of mine at McGill University. He admitted the young man and immediately started treatment.

Our patient recovered completely. He went back to high school, graduated with distinction, went to England, qualified as a barrister-at-law, and later accepted a diplomatic post in our Foreign Service. He has been, and continues to be, one of our most successful career diplomats, in many countries around the globe.

My Adventures as a District Medical Officer

In November 1952, the medical services in Siparia were experiencing a mini-crisis. The DMO there – a wartime refugee from Poland named Dr Michaelski – had resigned and was returning to his homeland. It seems that he was fed up with his practice, especially with the behaviour of some of the villagers. He had actually been put in court by one of them for some minor alleged offence. He was acquitted when the matter came up for hearing. I deduced, after meeting him, that he did not understand the psychology of the natives, and they did not understand his motives, which I am sure were quite respectable.

It is possible that I was sent to troublesome Siparia in order to educate me regarding the travails of the DMO, since I was very vocal in pointing to the shortcomings of at least one of them! At any rate, I was very pleased at this appointment: here was a chance for me to earn some money. I would be receiving my regular substantive salary and a travelling allowance. The Health Department would pay me a shilling for each infectious disease notification – and there were many of these around – and the legal department would pay me for each post mortem I performed. I would be allowed unlimited private practice and would be able to get medicines for my private patients, at almost a nominal cost, from the government dispensary.

For me, an added attraction was that I had lived for the first sixteen years of my life in that district, on a forty-eight acre cocoa estate. Indeed, by this time, my father had retired from teaching in San Fernando, and my parents had moved back to the estate.

My 'jurisdiction' covered some hundred square miles of interestingly varied geology, topography, industry, flora, fauna, people and dialect. There were Negroes, East Indians, Chinese, Portuguese, Caribs, Spaniards, English, French and numerous genetic mixtures of some, or many, of the above strains. The health offices under my control were situated in the following villages: Penal – named after the Spanish for 'pineapple' – Penal Rock Road ("by name and nature" as Dr Michaelski remarked, when I visited him before he left). Erin, where I myself spent my childhood and early youth – so christened by an early Irish Catholic missionary, Palo Seco – Spanish for 'dry stick', Oropouche – 'pocket of gold', Fyzabad, after a town in India, and at the hub, Siparia, an ancient Arawak settlement perched on a long plateau of sand from which, in the distance, the Gulf of Paria was visible.

Siparia was the headquarters of the district, and the 'capital' of the Ward of Siparia, boasting a court house, warden's office, police headquarters for the south-west of Trinidad, and a health centre, occupied by the medical officer for the entire county of St Patrick, the south-western peninsula, Dr Stella Abidh. This centre was located at the junction of the main road and Grell Street, named after the DMO who had lived in the adjoining quarters for several decades and who, as described earlier, I had met at the Port of Spain casualty department.

In this same residence I took up my abode in November 1952. The old wooden house was extremely comfortable: there were three large bedrooms, a huge living room, a kitchen and pantry, bathroom and lavatory, a wide corridor surrounding three-quarters of the building and from the outer banister to the roof, complete mosquito proofing. The eaves were wide, and doors opened from all the rooms to the corridor so that the entire building was quite dry and cool at all times, with no need for ventilating fans and, certainly no call for air-conditioning. Part of the corridor next to the front bedroom was partitioned off to form a small room, which was the examination room, and the contiguous corridor was the waiting room for private patients and for all emergencies, private or public, at night.

At the back of the building was an annexe, apparently intended as servants' quarters, but used as the residence for the ambulance driver, Thomas, and his family.

The evening after I arrived, a tall aristocratic looking negro gentleman and his white companion, knocked on my front door. They introduced themselves as Mr and Mrs Evan Rees. Mr Rees was the magistrate of the district, and the couple were my neighbours from across the road. This charming couple had come to pay their respects, and to welcome me to the district. We were fellow civil servants exiled at a remote outpost of the colony. They proffered their friendship, and offered to assist this lonely bachelor whenever he might be in need. I was greatly touched by this kind gesture. Mr Rees eventually became a High Court judge, and upon his retirement was appointed National Ombudsman.

My professional agenda was as follows:

7 a.m. to 9 a.m.	:	Private patients at home
9 a.m. to 12 noon	:	Health Office
12 noon to 1 p.m.	:	Lunch if not busy or on the road
1 p.m. to 4 p.m.	:	Health Office
4 p.m. to 6 p.m.	:	Private patients at home

At the Health Offices, the routine was as follows: inspection of vaccinations against smallpox done the week before, and signing the certificates of successful scratches. Next, I did the new vaccinations and repeats of those which were unsuccessful. These were rare, as the lymph we used from Connaught Laboratories of Canada was of very high potency. These were supplied by the Government Medical Stores in Port of Spain, and the 'cold chain' was strictly observed during storage and transport. The babies' reaction to the tiny, single scratch was varied: I was sure I could predict from their facial responses and the absence or nature, of their crying, how sensitive or stoic would be their personalities when they grew up!

In the days of Dr Grell, such high quality manufactured lymph was not available and the procedure was to take a drop from a recent vesicle and apply it to the new candidate. AIDS did not exist in those days. This homegrown material was not very reliable, so that the doctors of that era scratched at several sites – usually three in the hope that at least one would 'take'. Each doctor followed his own unique artistry: Dr Grell's, as my own arm testifies, drew an equilateral triangle, each side about five centimetres long. I have seen vertical rows and horizontal rows, reflecting perhaps the psychological idiosyncrasies of the respective practitioners. Vertically up – ambitious? Vertically down – depressive? Horizontal – complacent?

Next, I saw all the sick babies, prescribed for them, and the mothers passed along to the pharmacist, Mr Lewis, who travelled with his wares, by the district ambulance, and was generally able to set up shop before the DMO arrived. After these, I saw the old and elderly, then the younger ones and finally those who were not acutely ill, but awaiting examination for assessment of chronic conditions in order to be eligible for government relief.

Very shortly after my arrival in Siparia, I was awakened at about two in the morning by the telephone. It was the police, who told me that there had been a fatal motor accident on Mosquito Creek, and having informed Dr Mejias they were told by him that it was not in his jurisdiction but in that of the DMO for Siparia. I journeyed to the spot – a two mile long stretch infamous for motor accidents – and it occurred to me that it was on the far side of the Godineau River, which would place it in the County of Victoria – Dr Mejias' territory. In the event, I viewed the body of the victim, made my notes, and ordered its removal to my little mortuary situated in the Siparia Cemetery.

Later, I rechecked the boundaries on my map and confirmed that the body belonged to my San Fernando colleague. I have often wondered if the middle-aged doctor knew this and decided that he was in no mood to get out of bed at that ungodly hour or if he wished to pass on the $20 fee to young, impecunious, Dr Sampath!

I had heard stories of the reverse action by some DMOs who had allegedly dragged bodies across boundary lines into their own district!

My experience at the hospital stood me in good stead in the district, and the value of personally knowing the hospital doctors who would be attending to the patients I sent in, proved to be of great assistance to the patients. It was as if both the receiving doctor and I had a joint personal interest in the welfare of the sick person. For my part, I preferred to treat things like injuries myself, instead of burdening my already overworked colleagues with tasks which did not require in-patient care. In connection with this, the following article prepared by me was published in the *Civil Service Review* of December 1952.

The Civil Service Doctor

In undertaking to treat the sick members of the public, and to preserve the well being of the healthy, Government has, on its hands, a task which is as delicate as it is vital.

A sick person expects and deserves to be treated, not only with skill and competence, but also with patience, tact and courtesy. These virtues can be exhibited only by individuals who have the satisfaction of knowing that their efforts are appreciated by those to whom they minister. In Trinidad today, we are grieved to find that the government doctor and his patients are among the most dissatisfied members of the public.

The conditions of work for many doctors in the civil service are so unattractive that Government has found it impossible for at least the past ten years, and certainly today, to recruit enough doctors to fill the vacancies which exist in most branches of the health service. This shortage is most keenly felt in the hospitals, for these are the estuaries where all the streams of ill health and many of the rivers of poverty finally converge.

Here a small band of doctors are obliged to do the work of many, during long and tedious periods of time – occasionally thirty-two consecutive hours – without the possibility of compensating time off. So great is the crush of patients that some in the casualty departments may wait many hours for medical attention, and persons attending the out-patients' clinic may be forced to wait several months for their surgical treatment.

Hence, both doctor and patient remain dissatisfied. For his unfortunate plight, the patient commonly blames the doctor: the doctor is meanwhile aware that the patient (who is the doctor's master) neither knows, nor cares to know, how much the doctor must suffer in silence.

This point of contact, between an inefficient health service and an unhealthy public, is highly charged with human emotions, and the result of occasional explosions are commonly reported in our daily newspapers, much to the delight of those who revel in coarse sensationalism.

What are the reasons for this shortage of doctors in the Civil Service? A doctor in hospital begins at a salary of $300 per month, and after ten years service may receive $520. A doctor who has established himself, after a few months, in private practice, may earn $1,000 to $4,000 per month. In the face of this disparity, it is obvious why such a small percentage of doctors remain in hospital for more than eighteen months. We would be naive to consider that Government is unaware of these facts, yet, they consider this status to be immutable. This is not so: patients are thrown into the arms of private practitioners in such swarms because of the gross inadequacy of the government health service and the insufficiency of preventive medicine, especially in the fields of nutrition and parasitology. It would be only fair at this juncture to point out that the inefficiency of preventive medicine in Trinidad is due more to factors outside the compass of the public health section, for example, economic stress and a sadly disorientated agricultural policy, than intrinsic deficiencies.

Some of the intrinsic shortcomings are limited funds and a shortage of doctors in these fields. Here we are, confronted with an amazing double paradox: thousands of dollars are saved each year on the estimates for personal emoluments (doctors' salaries) because there are insufficient doctors to be paid, yet all the while, doctors who are constantly asking for salaries more consistent with their extra burdens and responsibilities, are refused their demands. Again, there is neither enough money nor enough doctors (in spite of the savings) to tackle such problems as hookworm and anaemia more intensively – problems which cost the government many thousands when the victims of these are admitted into hospital.

Doctors in hospitals are expected to perform their arduous tasks as a 'service to humanity'. It is said that doctors are 'not just civil servants', they are 'professional men' and should not equate their outlook with that of the civil service clerk. This attitude towards hospital doctors is mildly insane. Why, in the name of all that is fair, should any section of the civil service be expected to work considerably harder than any other similarly paid group? Surely it is reasonable to expect that the more exacting the work, the greater should be the financial reward.

A logical application of the policy of government with regard to overtime work in the civil service would at once preserve the unity of the service and give the doctor just recompense for his arduous and highly specialised labour. It has been estimated that a Grade 'C' medical officer works sixty hours per week, every week of the year. His overtime could be commuted to, say, eighty hours per month. Medical officers of Grades 'B' and 'A' also work considerable overtime and this could, likewise, be commuted and compensated for.

Hospital doctors have been doing this overtime work for many decades – on Sundays, public holidays and on fête days and nights. It is sad to reflect that not only an unfeeling public, but also their thoughtless colleagues in the civil service, have permitted such effort to go unrewarded for so long.

Viewing the general question of the service of health to the people on these islands in perspective, there emerges the impression that the District Medical Service is the crux of the problem. There are too few district medical officers and the district allocated to each is consequently too extensive and unwieldy. As a result, district medicine and minor surgery lack the efficiency and vitality they ought to possess. The present writer finds it difficult to follow the logic of government when it established the policy of appointing contract officers to the posts of DMO and requiring that hospital doctors should resign from the service, thereby losing their accrued advantages, if they wished to accept such contracts. One of the incentives which formerly kept many a doctor in the service – especially those psychologically equipped for general practice – was the hope that he might at some time be appointed as a DMO and, yet, remain in the service. The contract system has destroyed this incentive.

It is generally accepted that doctors who have spent some years in local hospitals make more efficient DMOs than those who have not, and hospital casualty officers, as well as consultants, have noticed that ex-hospital DMOs send in fewer cases requiring minor surgery, or a moderate degree of diagnostic acuity and therapeutic acumen, than do their non-hospital colleagues.

The abolition of the contract system, and the more widespread appointment of hospital doctors to DMO posts, would achieve three desirable results:

(a) It would attract more doctors to the service.
(b) It would reduce the burden on the hospitals.
(c) It would perpetuate an apparent and real sense of integration between patient, district and hospital, both before and after hospitalisation.

A further development, arising naturally out of this, would be the facility for DMOs to take up refresher appointments at the hospitals for six months of each three years. The resulting benefits which would thereby accrue to the standard of treatment of district patients would obviously be tremendous. The service would also gain in total strength and in practical mobility: at a moment's notice, any DMO would be able to fill any of the posts at a hospital, and a hospital doctor, of a few years' standing, any district post in the colony.

The civil servant is the servant of the public. Under the present scheme of organisation, the civil service doctor cannot serve his public efficiently, and the public is painfully and often embarrassingly aware of this.

To reorganise, for greater efficiency, will require courage and vigour. There are indications that these attributes are not entirely absent from the health department.

The practical value of some of the mundane chores, which as medical students we were required to perform at the Leeds General Infirmary, became apparent when I had to suture emergency incised and lacerated wounds in the district, with no nurse around. We students had the job of shaving that part of the patient which constituted the operation area. In the interest of delicacy, the male students did the men and the female students did the women. We objected strenuously – to no avail. "Are we training to be barbers or doctors?" we asked.

The cynical, if truthful, reply was, "Remember that the first surgeons were barbers!"

I became so adept at shaving – with the long 'cut-throat' razor to boot – that after one such session in Leeds the patient took me for a professional barber and invited me to give him a haircut after his operation!

As DMO, I was in great demand for social and sporting occasions: to give lectures, to bowl the first ball, and to be the judge at public speaking contests and athletic events. I once got the volleyball over the net after the third try. Who would have thought that I would be a star volleyball player for the Villeray ammunition team in Montreal during World War II, as part of my summer vacation employment from McGill University? *Sic transit gloria...* I once even took a team of youths on a photographic expedition, and later demonstrated how to develop and print the black and white film we exposed on the trip. I made many friends in Siparia: the greatest compliment paid to me was from an elderly lady who told me that I reminded her of Dr Jesse Grell!

The work was varied and interesting, and the private practice lucrative (by hospital standards), but extremely tiring, what with travelling hundreds of miles to and from health offices, viewing dead bodies, attending court and waking at night for emergencies at my residence and at private homes. One day, a patient saw me stretching my back, arms and legs, and she remarked that I appeared to be tired and sore. I replied in the affirmative and she thereupon gave me a firm but gentle rub on the back – a familiarity which I would normally have resented.

She appeared to be sympathetic, rather than forward, and to tell the truth, I rather enjoyed her expert touch. She asked whether I would like her to give me a massage that evening after work. I assumed that she was a professional masseuse and I accepted her offer. That evening it was the most wonderful massage I had ever had and when she was finished, I enquired her fee. She frowned and was obviously offended. She was not doing it for the money. She gave me regular massages after this, throughout my seven month stay in Siparia. She had a son and no husband and worked to support herself and her little boy. She accepted no gifts of any sort from me, but I attended to her and her son free of charge whenever they were ill.

It was here that I met my present spouse. The circumstances are related in my political book, *Search and Destroy*, and do not need to be repeated here.

Although I was appointed to act for six months in Siparia, seven months had passed before I was ordered back to San Fernando, and my colleague, Dr Percival Harnarayan, came to Siparia. It seemed that part of my published recommendation was being adopted! My income naturally reverted to a small fraction of what I had earned during my seven month bonanza, and the lure of filthy lucre impelled me to apply for a permanent DMO posting. I was informed, after three months at the hospital, that I would be appointed DMO Cedros, a district seventy miles from Port of Spain on the south-west tip of the St Patrick peninsula and seven miles from Venezuela. It was also thirty miles from Siparia, where my girlfriend and future spouse resided! There was good reason for this posting: most first appointments were for remote areas and officers were shifted after a year or two to more urbanised – and more lucrative – areas, so that after about ten years, they would be settled in or near the city, or large towns. Siparia would be one of these and ten years seemed much too long. I decided therefore to resign from the government service and put up my shingle in Siparia.

Private Medical Practice

For many decades, there were only two doctors in Siparia. When I was a boy, these were Dr Grell, the DMO, and Dr Hamilton J. Marcelin, an entirely private practitioner who lived at Moruga, some twenty miles away. Incidentally, it was here that Columbus's men landed in 1498 to draw fresh water after their leader had sighted the Trinity Hills and named the island 'La Trinidad'. Dr Marcelin was a fair-skinned mixture of Negro and French – by appearance in a ratio of about one to six. He was a descendant of French planters, who were given lands by the Spanish administration over a hundred years before. Dr Marcelin travelled from Moruga through forests, which still exist today, along the Penal Rock Road. Sick persons in the villages along his route would put out a flag when they needed his medical assistance. He would make his numerous house calls, prepare the appropriate medicines when he got to his Siparia office, and drop them off at the correct homes on his way back to Moruga at eventide. As a child, I and members of my family often availed ourselves of this extremely convenient and courteous arrangement.

When Dr Marcelin gave up his Moruga residence and his Siparia practice and moved both of these to San Fernando, residents of the 'Sand City' enjoyed the services only of the DMO until Dr Lloyd Jorsling started practice alongside his father's pharmacy, the Success Drug Store. Lloyd was my colleague and friend when I was DMO in his district, and he told me how grateful he was that, unlike my predecessor, I was interested in carrying on a vibrant private practice. It appears that he was inundated with patients, and the stress and strain of long hours at the office – sometimes from six in the morning to ten at night – was taking a toll on his mental and physical health. Now, in 1954, with three doctors in the village and all of them interested in private practice, life was much more comfortable for us all.

My father was in Siparia one day in 1953, when he suffered a massive heart attack. Lloyd kept him alive and phoned me at the hospital. I took my father in by ambulance, but the infarct was too widespread and he survived for only a month.

I lived with my mother, Amelia, and eldest sister, Annabelle, on our cocoa estate at the six and a quarter mile post on Penal Rock Road. I held a little morning office – usually two or three patients only – and then journeyed, accompanied by my sister, who agreed to be my receptionist without pay until my practice began to make some money. My little Hillman Minx performed brilliantly. In January 1954, the massive scarlet and orange blossoms of the huge Immortelle trees brightened our early morning trips, and in February and March, these gave way to the scintillating gold of the Poui. Occasionally, patients would stop me along the route and like Dr Marcelin – but without the flag, which I did not encourage – I would make instantaneous house calls. While most of these were non-emergency matters, I was fortunate enough to pass by in time to save two babies. Their mothers had been in labour overnight, dilation was complete, but they would not emerge, and the attending local midwife – the *chamaine* – was unable to extract them. One had a prolapsed umbilical cord and the other's shoulders were stuck transversely. With the simplest of manoeuvres, I was able to let them emerge. Today I remember these babies, now over forty years old, every time I pass their parents' homes. These people were Brahmins – the highest caste of Hindus – and it seemed to me to be the height of irony that childbirth practice in such a sensitive area would be entrusted to a person of one of the lowest castes. *Chamaine* is the feminine of *chamar* – an untouchable. The duties of this midwife involved not only dealing with the lower part of the human body, but what could be the most unclean, and also with cleaning those areas and the linen involved. For a very long time, very few Hindu girls applied to the hospitals for training to be nurses and midwives.

When my practice started, and for one year afterwards, I lived at my mother's home, eleven miles away. Early in 1955, I was able to acquire half an acre of land about a quarter of a mile from my office. I built a house on it and moved in. I started a small after-hours emergency office at my residence and my workload increased tremendously. My weekday hours were eight in the morning to six in the evening. On Sundays and Public Holidays, I attended at my main office, officially from eight in the morning to midday, but more often than not, I could not get home for lunch until two in the afternoon. For a short period, I cut out the Sunday and holiday main office visits, but this proved to be a disaster: patients came to my house in droves and I had to manage without the help of a receptionist, dispensing assistant and the previous records of those regulars who came to me. I quickly reverted to the former arrangement.

London Interlude

In 1956, I decided that I would do a postgraduate course in ophthalmology. My younger brother, Hugh, was in his final year in medicine at Oxford, and I was hoping that he would take over my general practice. I took a large loan from Barclays Bank, and purchased a lovely house at Bayshore, on the waterfront, a few miles from Port of Spain. I planned to set up residence and a practice in ophthalmology there. I let my Siparia house, and loaned my practice to a colleague, Dr Noble Sarkar, who had been with me at McGill, and was actually in my platoon in the Canadian Officers' Training Corps during World War II. He, like me, had studied medicine in England on a Colonial Welfare and Development scholarship. He and Dr Simon Ramesar had been at Sheffield.

On the plane out of Piarco, Trinidad, I was seated next to an Englishwoman, who appeared to be upper middle class and quite sophisticated. She seemed to be in her forties. After a polite exchange of identities, she asked if I had ever been to England before, and whether it was for a visit. I revealed that I had trained in her country, and also how hospitable I had found the people to be. She warned me that things had changed radically since the defeat of the Nazis; that I would be sorely disappointed if I expected the same kind of reception when I arrived: that the British were rather more intolerant and resentful of 'strangers', and that there was substantial intensification of racial prejudice and hostility.

Before World War II, colonials visiting Britain were mainly students who presented no economic threat, and were of an intellectual and social standard which made them exotically attractive to Britishers. During the War, the influx of colonial non-white soldiers and airmen was enthusiastically welcomed by a nation fighting for her very survival, but after the War, most colonial immigrants were economic refugees seeking a livelihood, in close competition with the locals. These 'invaders' were largely from the underprivileged masses in their own countries, and occasionally some of their ethical and moral standards left a great deal to be desired. These were the days of Enoch Powell's call for the repatriation of non-whites *en masse*, of the graffiti on the walls of Bayswater 'Keep the Water White', and at a medical convention, a call from the floor for stopping non-white doctors from disembarking at Heathrow!

It may or may not be significant that after about an hour in her seat, my Englishwoman disappeared, and I travelled to London with the seat next to mine vacant!

My year at Moorfield's Eye Hospital and the Institute of Ophthalmology was uneventful. My brother, Hugh, and I exchanged visits almost every weekend. He already had a Masters degree in Anthropology, from McGill, before he came to medical school, and he decided to take up Psychiatry – a logical step. So that, despite my Diploma in Ophthalmology, for me, the eyes would not have it all, since, I was uninclined to leave the general practice which I had built up so strenuously and embark on what would be the start of another practice.

Back to General Practice

I returned to Trinidad in 1957. My political party, the People's National Movement, had won the general elections on a platform of anti-colonialism and independence. I resumed my general practice at Siparia, and also assumed the appointment as part-time ophthalmologist at the General Hospital, San Fernando, as it was now called, the name 'Colonial' being anathema to the new nationalist dispensation – but the change in name changed its nature not a whit.

By this time, there were several other doctors in Siparia, in Penal five miles away and in Fyzabad four miles off. The work load was much less, and I spent a great deal of time in political activity. I was a candidate of the PNM, for the county of St Patrick, for the parliament of the ill-fated Federation of the West Indies. My rivals for the seat were Tubal Uriah Buzz Butler (whose lieutenant had returned with me on the SS *Matina*, in 1950) and my former Scoutmaster, Mohammed Shah, of the 5th Naparima Scout Group. My scoutmaster won the seat. After my defeat, I retired from active politics, and spent most of my non-medical time writing for the local press on political, economic and sociological matters, and serving on several government committees and a Commission of Enquiry into the Prevalence of Race and Colour Discrimination. Some of these activities are recorded in my publication, *Half Slave Half Free*, 1971.

By 1973, I was greatly disillusioned with the PNM and its leader, Dr Eric Williams, and I resigned from the party hoping to relinquish political activity forever. But the economic plight of the country, and the disgraceful treatment meted out by Dr Williams to his conscientious and competent deputy, Mr A.N.R. Robinson, whose only crime was to seek the economic welfare of the masses of the population, drew me once more into active politics. After this, my articles in the press became stridently critical of Prime Minister

Williams and his government, and I joined Mr Robinson in his new party, the Democratic Action Congress.

From 1950 to the present, I have been active in the Trinidad and Tobago Branch of the British Medical Association which, after our national independence, changed its name – but not its nature! – to the Trinidad and Tobago Medical Association. Subsequent chapters will deal with these activities.

My political activities did not interfere with my medical work: for one thing, the ten doctors now present in the five mile radius around Siparia made the individual load lighter, and provided adequate facilities to patients during my absence in the evenings and at night. My medical colleagues, with whom I have always had an excellent relationship, have been most cooperative at all times. But, when I was at home during the night, I began to find patients' demands very disturbing and jolting to my equanimity. I was simply getting older, and couldn't stand the strain. It was exasperating in 1980 (when it hardly mattered in 1950), to be awakened from sleep several times during the night: it was intolerable to be disturbed during the most intimate of biological functions. And this occurred, ante- and anti-climactically, with such frequency, that I pondered on ways to end it. In discussing this with some of my colleagues, l learned that some of them simply instructed a member of the family to tell the caller that, "the doctor is not at home". One doctor's long-suffering spouse, on telling the caller this, was asked, "But, how then can I see his car in the garage?" Despite the heat of the moment, she promptly responded, "One of his friends picked him up." But such deception, even to save my sanity, was not part of my moral code – however lax it may be in other respects – so I decided that if I wished to reach the biblical three score and ten, I would have to live elsewhere, and travel daily to my office. My mother had sold the Penal Rock Road property, but had inherited a seventeen acre block, at La Romaine, from her own mother, Agnes Lucky. I bought this land from my mother, sold a five acre plot to my spouse, who erected a fine building on it, and we and our family moved into this home in June 1980.

My political activities from 1980 to 1991 were full and exciting. I was very active in the formation and further activities of the 'Accommodation', an amalgamation of political parties in opposition to the government, and was, at different times, Treasurer and

Research Officer of the party which evolved from this coalition – the National Alliance for Reconstruction. This political party went on to defeat the ruling PNM by thirty-three seats to three, and formed the new government in 1986.

Although I served as Chairman of the Agricultural Development Bank, as Deputy Chairman of the Caroni Sugar and industrial complex, and as a member of the Committee investigating State Enterprises – all very important and time consuming undertakings – I never allowed these activities to interfere with my regular medical practice. I served in parliament as a government senator, but declined the Prime Minister's request that I should accept a ministerial post, because I would then have had to retire from medical practice.

*

In the following pages, I relate some of the experiences I had during the course of my medical practice. In retrospect, I find some of them very amusing, and I trust that some of my readers will also share in this reaction.

Evidence in Court

A doctor's evidence in court is very important, and is often vital in determining culpability and final sentencing, when someone is charged and when convicted. Yet, for a busy doctor, it is something of a nuisance. Not only does absence from his work involve financial loss for the private practitioner, especially when the matter is heard many miles away from his office, but, for both the government paid and the patient paid medico, the cross-examination by the opposition is often quite rigorous, cruel, and occasionally extremely lengthy and loaded with innuendo and irrelevancy. Aspersions are often cast on the competence, integrity and veracity of the doctor. In one instance at Siparia, when I gave evidence of the injuries sustained by a young man who was allegedly beaten up by the police, the police attorney cross-examined me for *three hours*! As it happened, the police were eventually found guilty.

The importance of writing accurate and detailed notes, and not just general descriptions of injuries found, was driven home to me by the following incident which occurred when I was at the Port of Spain casualty department.

Six wounded men were brought in at about ten one Saturday night. I attended to each in turn – one of them, with a deep abdominal puncture, died on the examination couch. It had been a family and neighbourly fight, and knives had been used all around. When they had all been attended to and disposed of – three discharged, two to the wards, and one to the mortuary – the policeman in attendance handed me their record book, in which details were not required – only general statements as to the nature and seriousness of the wounds (danger to life). The doctor's immediate opinion often determined the gravity of the charges and the matter of bail.

Opposite the names of the patients listed, I wrote 'Multiple stab wounds', and for the admitted patients and the dead man, (perceptively!) 'Dangerous to life'. When the case came up for hearing the following year in Port of Spain, I journeyed from San Fernando, forty miles away, and, on arrival at the court, I was called into conference by the defence attorney and the crown prosecutor, both eminent King's Counsels (Elizabeth II became Queen only in 1952). They wished to save this young inexperienced doctor the embarrassment of going into the witness box, and giving evidence contrary to that of the post mortem finding of a single stab wound. They suggested that my entry in the police book of "Multiple stab wounds" could be interpreted to mean that the blade, having gone through several layers of tissue including the intestine, did, in fact, constitute "Multiple" wounds!

It was an ingenious piece of reasoning. It would save my face, but I decided that I would go into the box, and tell the whole story exactly as it happened that night. The fatherly judge was very sympathetic, and agreed that, in the circumstances, my error was easily pardonable. This is a lesson which I have never forgotten, and it has stood me in good stead.

(As a flattering aside, at a social gathering, the President of the Republic, Mr Noor Hassanali, a High Court judge, who had occasionally sat for cases of wounding in which I gave evidence, told the Prime Minister, Mr A.N.R. Robinson, in my presence, how impressed he was by the accuracy of my descriptions of injuries sustained by persons I had examined!)

Caught Speeding

On the morning of 13th July 1951, as doctor in charge of the maternity department at the San Fernando hospital, I was waiting for one of my patients to dilate fully. It was her first pregnancy and her pains were variable in intensity and frequency. It was a matter for watchful anticipation. At about nine-fifty, the telephone rang. I was required to attend court, at Chaguanas, immediately – it was about fifteen miles away – to give evidence in a wounding case. I got the notes and hurried along to my faithful Hillman Minx – thirty-two miles to the gallon, with a speed up to eighty miles per hour – and sped away. I promptly got caught in a speed trap on the Couva long stretch, just four miles from the court.

After the case was heard, I told the prosecuting Inspector of Police what had happened. A few days later, I received the following, delivered to me personally by the policeman who usually brought to doctors their summons to attend court:

TRINIDAD POLICE FORCE

..........Headquarters..........Police Station.

..........25th..........day of ....July..........19.5.1.

CAUTIONARY NOTICE

It has been reported to me that at..10.35..a.m./p.m. on the ....13th..........

day of ....July..........19.5.1.

at(..Cunupia Main Road.. - ..C. Anetta:..........you were found

to have been the driver of a certain motor vehicle to wit motor car P.B.2916 and that you did drive the said vehicle at a speed greater than permitted in relation to such class of vehicle, to wit 57 M.P.H., contrary to Chap. 16: 1 Sec. 44 (C)

Having considered the facts I have decided to refrain from proceeding in court, but to issue this Cautionary Notice instead, and to warn you that any further offence will lead to a summons being issued against you.

....
Superintendent of Police

..........Caroni's..........Division

To : Dr. Martin Sampath

..........32 Coffee St. San F'do.

G.P., Tr./To.—1422—3M—8/49

Incidentally, I got back to the ward in time to deliver the baby, who will never know how the speed of the doctor on the open road, and the lack of it in his cosy cocoon, resulted in our almost simultaneous rendezvous at the appointed place.

Left? Right? Or No Side At All?

I once examined and sutured several cutlass chops on the arm, forearm and hand of a man, while he was lying on the casualty couch with an intravenous drip on the other arm. I sent him to the ward for further treatment. When the matter came up for hearing, both the ward surgeon and I were called to give medical evidence. The surgeon testified an hour before me. Our notes were on opposite sides of the same record card. Lo and behold, when I looked at the surgeon's notes I discovered, to my embarrassment, that he had described the wounds as being on the right limb, while my record stipulated the left! The astute defence lawyer had determined, beyond all doubt, that the victim had no injuries whatsoever on his left limb and, from evidence based on my notes, his right limb was unscathed. The K.C. then put it to the jury that medical evidence proved conclusively that the man had no injuries at all! The jury did not buy that logic, and the assailant was found guilty and sent to jail.

I am told that, after we doctors left the court, the scars were demonstrated to the jury, but they never told us whose anatomical orientation was wrong that time.

A Legal Fiction

It is customary, on direct examination, for a lawyer to ask a doctor giving expert evidence, "Do you remember the night of [say] 20th March 1952?" The doctor does not remember if that night ever existed, and has absolutely no recollection of what, where or to whom he did anything. But, he has been called to give specific evidence, justice demands that he speaks with direct knowledge and memory, he has in his hands the notes he made at the time in his own handwriting, and the court, and all persons within, accept that he is able to 'refresh his memory' by looking at those notes; so he lies and answers, "Yes, sir", and everybody is happy with this universal acceptance of a legal fiction.

Attorney:
"On that night do you remember attending to one John Smith?"

Doctor:

(Looking at the name on the top of his patient's card): "Yes, Sir."

Attorney:

"Do you see him in court today?"

The doctor, (looking around and seeing several persons who could be John Smith, and everyone except the doctor knows which one is Smith, so the doctor feels like a fool, but, with great presence of mind, notices one of them in the correct place for victims), answers "Yes," and points him out. The doctor keeps up this legal fiction because after all, the play's the thing.

Many a time have I entered my ward in the morning, after a busy day, followed by an eventful night, and seen a patient whom I had treated in casualty, and admitted during the night, and not only do I not recognise the patient by name, nor by features, but do not remember having attended to him. On looking at my notes, I realise that I had made the correct diagnosis, and had treated and prescribed for him correctly. Several of my colleagues have had the same experience. We had been mere automatons, reduced to that state by sheer fatigue, our sanity protected by a dissociation of our memory centres from the rest of our brain. Luckily for our patients, the recall of our training, and our physical skill, remained fully active. But, perhaps not alert enough to distinguish right from left!

A general practitioner once boasted, to a group of younger colleagues, that he had thirty years of medical experience. One of his listeners remarked, unkindly, "You mean that you have had one year's experience thirty times?"

There is a great deal of truth in the youngster's statement: general practice can be almost the same from year to year, and would be quite boring if the patients themselves, as opposed to their ailments, did not possess such varied personalities, and did not react in so many different ways to the doctor and to his treatment. But, as if to add a little condiment to his practice, there do appear, from time to time, some interesting and some unusual situations which make general practice worth pursuing. These are not necessarily difficult cases or matters requiring medical heroism, but interesting in their own right, nevertheless. Some of these are described later.

Respiratory ailments are the bread and butter of general practice, constituting perhaps 75% of practice. Out of these proceeds, the doctor feeds, clothes and educates his family. The other 25% of ailments, which involve every other part of the body and soul of his clients, provide the gravy – his luxuries, savings and investments for the period of his life when he can no longer earn a living.

The general practitioner's attitude towards his patients – the so-called bedside manner – is of profound importance: a 'nice' doctor's treatments always make his patients better faster, and so increase his clientele and his income. While such a statement may sound more cynical than clinical, the fact is, that a doctor who *obviously* identifies with the suffering of the patient, or in the case of a child, with the fears and misgivings of the parents, will be sought more often than the most clinically competent physician who appears to take merely a scientific interest in the patient's illness, assuming he is a reasonably competent doctor with reasonable fees.

Foreign Bodies

A child, in the course of the exploration of his or her orifices, will sometimes insert small objects or fragments, wherever they can be introduced, and occasionally the child cannot get them out again. I have extracted seeds – in Trinidad and Tobago these are usually corn (maize) and pigeon pea grains – beads, pieces of sponge, food, fruit and so on from the nostrils. Nothing is usually noticed until a foul smell develops, and the mother diagnoses this to be the result of a 'bad head cold', which their doctors are sometimes persuaded that it is, and treat with antibiotics and nose drops for weeks in some cases, with no positive result.

I extract the foreign body with a suitably curved hair pin, which I have named 'the magic weapon'. The one I have in my possession must have removed five hundred foreign bodies in its lifetime, and shows no sign of wear and tear. It has earned thousands of dollars, and pleased hundreds of mothers. It has been the most effective, cheapest and most lucrative instrument ever made.

From the ear, I have extracted foreign bodies with another hairpin of a different modification – just a one millimetre right-angle hook at the business end; but smooth objects such as beads have to be syringed out.

One baby came in with persistent coughing and vomiting. This was caused by a fragment of a blade of grass stuck in its pharynx, easily removed with forceps.

I often see young children with a variety of foreign bodies in their vaginas, presenting with a persistent vaginal discharge. In these cases, a finger in the rectum, gently stroking the vagina in front from back to front, usually gets the foreign body out.

A young lady of thirty-five came to me complaining of abdominal pain, gaseous distension and constipation for seven days. There had been no evacuative response to senna and salts and castor oil. On examination, I felt at my finger tip a peculiar mass in her rectum and, with a swab-holding forceps, I extracted a tightly matted mass of fibre followed, like an erupting volcano, by a week of pent-up alimentary magma.

This young lady, in response to the popular call for the ingestion of fibre, had eaten, at one sitting, ten mangoes of the 'vert' variety. This type of fruit, unlike others like 'Julie', 'Calabash', 'Graham' and 'Starch', has a very large number of long, fibrous strings attached to the seed, and usually the sweet, delicious pulp is sucked off the seed, leaving the fibre behind. She had eaten it in slices, fibre and all!

A child of six was brought to me complaining of watery, bloody stools and intense rectal pain on attempting to defecate. My index finger tip encountered an aggregation of sharp edged objects just within the rectal sphincter. One of these was extracted, and it turned out to be the flanged seed of a delicious cherry, which I knew very well; these fruits are chewed, seeds and all, but the seeds are not swallowed. Wild animals also know this, even cud-chewing beasts: my deer had their fill under my cherry tree, but they all spat out the seeds, in neat little heaps under the tree, after regurgitation. The little girl was in tremendous pain, and, after syringing in a little local surface anaesthetic, I removed over fifty of the seeds from the badly excoriated rectum. General and local antibiotics completed the treatment.

I have several times removed gauze packing from vaginas following dilation and curettege done elsewhere, and once even a condom! I advised the lady that she should request that her partner should use a more closely fitting one in future.

My most unusual vaginal foreign body was half of a lemon: the lady had been advised that lemon juice was indicated for maintaining the acidity of that organ, and she decided that reservoir therapy would fit the bill.

Metal splinters in the cornea, air gun pellets, broken needles, fragments of glass in the sole and so on I have removed by the hundred, but the unusual ones listed above have stuck amusingly in my memory.

Itching and Scratching

By far the commonest cause of itching of the skin, in Trinidad and Tobago, is scabies infestation. The Sarcoptes scabiei is endemic in our overcrowded primary schools; the children bring it home, and infect everyone there. In many instances, this condition remains undiagnosed for weeks, even months, and too often parents get all sorts of expensive creams, some containing steroids, from their friendly neighbourhood pharmacist, before coming to a diagnosing doctor. The standard treatment has never yet failed me: scrub the entire family with an antiseptic soap, dry the skin with a clean towel, apply benzyl benzoate or gammabenzene cream to all parts of every member, put on a sterile (boiled or ironed) set of clothing, and sleep on similarly treated bed clothes. Also, check each schoolchild regularly for re-infection. Secondary infections of the mites' burrows are extremely common, especially after steroids have been used, and I always, in these cases, supply an oral antibiotic.

Occasionally, the unfortunate child has already developed acute nephritis, following streptococcal infection of the burrows. These are actively treated accordingly.

When I was a boy, most primary school children in rural areas went barefoot, and infestation by the jigger or chigoe flea (Dermatophilius or Tonga penetrans) was widespread. The sweetest itch I have ever had was from such a creature in my foot. A very recent attack by a flea can be frustrated with a sharp needle, to remove the speck of animal life, but a twenty-four hour beach head is deep and difficult. After a few days, the egg sac has expanded to the size of a pea, and the entire animal is best extracted by working it loose from the surrounding tissue with a blunt needle, and taking it out whole, without rupturing the abdomen. A clean little hole is left, into which an antiseptic drop may be introduced. Should this gravid female be left in the skin, she shoots her eggs into the dust where her offspring lie in wait for the naked feet of our offspring. She then dies in situ, and the resulting festering sore has been the focus for tetanus infection, in some instances, and streptococcal nephritis in others.

Toes and fingers are the commonest sites of infestation, but the flea is no respecter of anatomy, and I have seen them in the eyelid, ear, buttock and penis.

With the advent of shoes, chigoe infestation has almost completely disappeared, and it is now such a rarity that its appearance anywhere is an occasion for a treatise in a medical journal.

As chigoes have gone, however, the vacant spaces between the toes have been occupied by another itch, namely athlete's foot.

Allergic Reactions

These are common and are sometimes life threatening. The appearance of weal-like lesions (urticaria) is called, in Trinidad and Tobago, 'mad blood', and affected patients are discomfited as much by this name as by the itching. At the time that I graduated from medical school in 1950, anti-histamines had just come into clinical use: the first was Parke Davis' Benadryl, and the standard treatment was the old adrenalin subcutaneous injection, plus the new Benadryl capsule every three or four hours. While working at the San Fernando hospital, I had been given a shot of Procaine Penicillin for a severe throat infection. The following night, I developed a massive urticaria with a violent flare at the injection site. My uncle, Dr Shadrack, gave me the standard treatment – quite successfully, but I felt pleasantly drunk, not pugnaciously or amorously, but tranquilisingly inebriated. I had been invited to have dinner that evening, and as the urticaria was under control, and my hosts were the parents of a close medical colleague of mine, I felt that I ought to keep the appointment. My friend had a lovely and gifted sister, just a few years younger than me. (It was broadly hinted that there could possibly have been a matrimonial future involved!)

I thoroughly enjoyed the dinner and the conversation, but the effect of the Benadryl was such that the very real charmer – flower-blushed unseen – its fragrance was wasted on me, and the lucky girl escaped my clutches, and eventually married someone much more deserving, and now has a wonderful husband and a group of happy, beautiful children. There have been – belatedly – many improved, long-acting, non-sedating anti-histamines since then.

I have had a few severe drug reactions among my patients and some minor ones, but fortunately no fatalities. The commoner agents have been penicillin, streptomycin, sulphas and, to my surprise, B12!

There commonly occur allergic manifestations in persons who are unable to pin-point the causative allergen, but very many, though not all, can be detected after close questioning and astute detective work on the part of the relatives, the patient and the doctor as catalyst.

An elusive egg reaction:

One woman came to me with an urticaria, after eating eggs. She told me that she commonly got this after eating eggs from her own yard fowls, but never from eggs she bought in the market three miles away. My explanation was that there must have been some plant or insect in her yard on which her birds fed, and to which she could have been allergic when these chemicals were transferred by the hens to their eggs.

A recurring lunchtime reaction:

In the days when I attended at my office on Sunday mornings, I was habitually sought by one of my regular patients – a young woman, of about thirty-five, who arrived regularly and punctually, as my receptionist was closing the office windows and I was packing my bag. On each occasion, her face, neck, arms and upper chest would be red, swollen and itching. The condition always responded to my standard treatment: Piriton intra-muscular and oral. I was always anxious at that hour to get home, in order to assuage a growling stomach and a low blood sugar, but after the fourth such visit I decided to try and find out what the external irritant could have been, since the eruption on exposed areas only suggested contact as the cause. So, after giving the injection, I asked her to tell me in detail, everything she had done just before the rash appeared.

"Well," she said, "after lunch, we all sat on the floor, watching television. That's all."

"Did you rub anything on your face and arms, any cream or lotion or anything?"

"No."

"Did any of your children or your husband hug you, or did you use a towel or scarf?"

"Not at all."

"Well then, did anything else happen, cigarette or cock-sec (anti-mosquito coil) smoke?"

"No. My son just took the swatter and killed a fly on the wall."

On hearing the word 'fly', my ears involuntarily pricked themselves up. A little bell rang in my head: "What sort of fly was it?"

"Actually it was a Jack Spaniard, there is a large nest under the eaves outside the window."

So that was the answer! She was allergic to the chemicals which emanated from these large red wasps, and she got the attacks every Sunday after lunch when she and her children congregated in front of their newly acquired television set, their movements, laughter and the sound of the noisy appliance made the insects restless, and they excitedly released the chemical to which my patient was allergic.

I had had a few patients who were allergic to this insect, and it was this experience which alerted me to the possibility that the 'fly' could have been a Jack Spaniard.

A contact skin test with a dead insect later confirmed the diagnosis.

One of the patients, dangerously allergic to the Jack Spaniard, has given me permission to mention his name and to report that he now chews and swallows a few leaves of the Neem plant every day, and this has cured his allergy to the wasp! He is Mr Sookram Gangadeen of Quarry Village, Siparia. The botanical name for the Neem plant is *Azadivachta Indica*. It is also a mosquito repellent.

Human Wetlands

In the humid tropics, skin fungi have a field day. The areas below the breasts, and the nappy regions, are their battlegrounds of choice. The major quislings of these invaders are the brassiere and the disposable diaper.

My professor of anatomy (whom we met in the early pages of this treatise), the New Zealander, in describing the anatomy and function of the platysma muscle, which runs from the neck to the breast, once told his class that in former times Maori women wore no brassieres, and that their breasts were amply supported by their platysmas. This muscle was so well developed, he said, that some of these ladies, instead of winking at you, would 'flick a tit for you'! In Trinidad and Tobago, I have never seen a breast intertrigo in any non-brassiered person, and there are numerous traditional East Indian dressers among my patients all non-brassiered and all non-intertriginous. I have seen very severe cases of this malady, which do not respond to the usual desiccating powders, but which resolve rapidly on anti-fungals, such as Mycostatin and the Conazoles. I also advise them to boil their brassieres, or pass a hot iron on them, and to stay without them as long as possible.

Incidentally, this symbol of female subjection has now appeared among the Maoris, as I discovered when visiting them in 1992, and the younger generation of East Indian women in Trinidad have also donned this anatomical disguise.

The incidence of very severe rashes in babies' groin and genital areas has reached alarming proportions: some of them become infected with bacteria, and inguinal glands are sometimes quite enlarged. There are mothers who are financially struggling to get food for their families, who have no disposable income, but who keep their babies in disposable diapers. Are they just too lazy to wash cloth diapers? Or have they fallen victim to the obscene advertisements which promote these accoutrements as desirable status symbols? These horrible lesions, when seen by me, are sometimes so badly infected and so raw, that I have to give a systemic antibiotic in addition to the local application of a fungicide, plus a weak steroid. The classic zinc and castor oil preparations are useless in these cases.

Pox, Malaria, Yellow Fever and Rabies

When I was acting as District Medical Officer for Siparia, I once saw a patient covered with pox. He had a high fever, and was in great distress. I diagnosed smallpox, and sent him to the Medical Officer of Health, Dr Stella Abidh, a very senior and experienced doctor. She sent me a note politely letting me know that she appreciated my diligence, but that the man had only chickenpox with secondarily infected vesicles. He was a diabetic. Although I had seen many old smallpox cases with badly scarred faces, there had not been an active case in Trinidad and Tobago for several decades, thanks to our compulsory vaccination regime. Today, no case of smallpox has been seen anywhere in the world – the virus does not appear to exist any more, except in laboratories where one or more unfortunate fatal episodes have been reported.

In my private practice, chickenpox epidemics are very common. In November 1977, I inadvertently scratched my right lower jaw, after examining a young girl who had chickenpox. I developed shingles (Herpes zoster) in the distribution of my right third cervical nerve, and eventually gave chickenpox to all the members of my family! It was Dr Pickles, working in an isolated valley in the north of Britain, who, by noticing the spread of these two conditions in his closed community, deduced that a single agent was responsible for both infections.

There is a belief widespread in Trinidad and Tobago that if the shingles on one side spreads to the other side, it will squeeze the victim in a fatal embrace. Paradoxically, this happens to be a very consoling dictum, for zoster is never bi-lateral. This knowledge has led many medical students into the error of believing that the name Herpes zoster cingularis is H.V. singulars, meaning a single nerve,

72

but, in fact, the derivation is from the Latin 'cingula', meaning a belt or band.

Most patients are very worried about the duration and results of this sometimes excruciatingly painful infection, so I show them a photograph of myself taken at its height – the fifth day – and tell them that it is a ten day self-limiting disease. When I then show them my own face and chest, their anxiety, and a great deal of the physical pain, appear immediately to vanish! This also bolsters their confidence in my simple treatment: Paracetamol tablets, Caladryl cream and Phenobarbitone tablets at night. Anti-viral drugs may have a place, but they are at present too expensive for my patients. Zovirax was not known in 1977, or I would have used it for my own infection! I seldom prescribe it, but it appears to be most effective when used very early, and may prevent or alleviate post herpetic neuralgia.

Malaria was very common when I was a boy. I got repeated attacks, and during my bouts of high fever, my hallucinations took the form of travelling at great speed in gigantic loops from planet to planet! I must have been between seven and nine at that time, and knew about stars and planets, but Buck Rogers and other inter-planetary comic book heroes were unknown, and I don't think I had yet read H.G. Wells and Jules Verne. So in my imagination, I was a space traveller, long before such journeys became a reality or even commonplace fiction.

My father always kept a stock of quinine sulphate powder and a good supply of gelatin capsules, each calibrated for the appropriate dosage. Although the malaria vector – the Anopheles mosquito is still with us, the malaria protozoon – the Plasmodium is absent, and those cases which crop up from time to time are recent arrivals from Africa, or India or Venezuela. Routine blood smears occasionally showed the Plasmodium in the early 1950s, when I still worked at the hospitals, and I treated patients for malaria until about 1960, but few proven cases have been found among the local population from then to this day.[3] This has been the result of sustained liquidation of the parasite by drugs, but the reduction of the mosquito population by regular spraying of their habitats has not been successful.

---

[3] In late 1994, about a dozen cases re-appeared in a particular locality in Trinidad.

Dogs, Bats and Rabies

During the 1920s and 1930s, in Trinidad, a mysterious disease, causing paralysis in farm animals, reached epidemic proportions. Dr Lennox Pawan, a local pathologist, discovered the Negri bodies of rabies in the brains of our Desmodus rufus bats: the bats were biting the animals at night, in the dark, and drinking their blood. They contracted the fatal disease from those bites. Now, in some other countries, rabies is generally contracted through the bites of rabid canines, mainly dogs, wolves and foxes. We see and treat very many dog bites in Trinidad and Tobago, but no case of rabies has ever been found in a dog or in any of its victims. One of the persisting nightmares of our doctors, is that one day, a rabid bat may bite some dogs, and produce a canine reservoir of rabies, with the human population at risk. This apprehension is compounded by the fact that one of our wild animals, the manicou or opposum, and some fruit-eating bats have been found to harbour the virus. Incidentally, our local name 'manicou' is the French patois for 'main en queue' – a hand in the tail - a reference to the prehensile capacity of the animal's caudal appendage.

Yellow Fever and the Red Howler Monkey

I have witnessed three yellow fever epidemics in Trinidad. These occur at intervals of ten to fifteen years. Human fatalities have been very few. The epidemics have been among the Red Howler monkey population of our forests. Every decade and a half, or thereabouts, dead monkeys are found in substantial numbers by our hunters, and the Yellow Fever virus has been found in their blood. Apparently, it takes about fifteen years for a critical susceptible population of monkeys to accrue. In the forest, the vector is the Haemagogus mosquito, which breeds in the water that collects in the saprophytic wild pines adorning the branches of our trees. Human victims have been hunters who have been bitten by these infected insects. Now, in our urban and built-up areas, the Aedes aegypti mosquito breeds in the clear water of discarded pots and pans which abound in our country, and as this species of mosquito is the vector of Yellow Fever in other countries, a fear is that some day our domestic Aedes will stray near to the forest, take a liking to the blood of an infected Red Howler, and bring the disease into our human population. Thankfully, while many thousands of the Aedes have been captured and examined for the virus, there has been not a single positive so far. As a precaution, mass inoculations have been and are carried out constantly, and our country is deemed free of Yellow Fever. Incidentally, we have Dengue Fever epidemics each year, on account of the continued breeding of the Aedes which is also its vector.

My spouse and I had a mildly irritating experience in connection with this: by World Health Organisation protocol, a Yellow Fever inoculation is considered to be effective for ten years, starting seven days after the inoculation. A re-inoculation, before the ten year period has ended, is deemed to be effective immediately for another ten years, but, if that time has elapsed, any re-inoculation is deemed to be a new inoculation, and is again effective only after seven days. In September 1983, we left Trinidad for Nairobi, with valid inoculations recorded in our little yellow books, but ten years had just expired while we were in Kenya. We were booked to go to Bombay after the Conference, on a certain day, and, as we had to be re-inoculated, it meant that we had to re-route our trip through Seychelles and Sri Lanka in order to use up seven days before entering India! Incidentally, if we had gone to India directly from Trinidad, we would have had no need for a Yellow Fever inoculation, since Trinidad, in spite of our Red Howlers, is deemed Yellow Fever free!

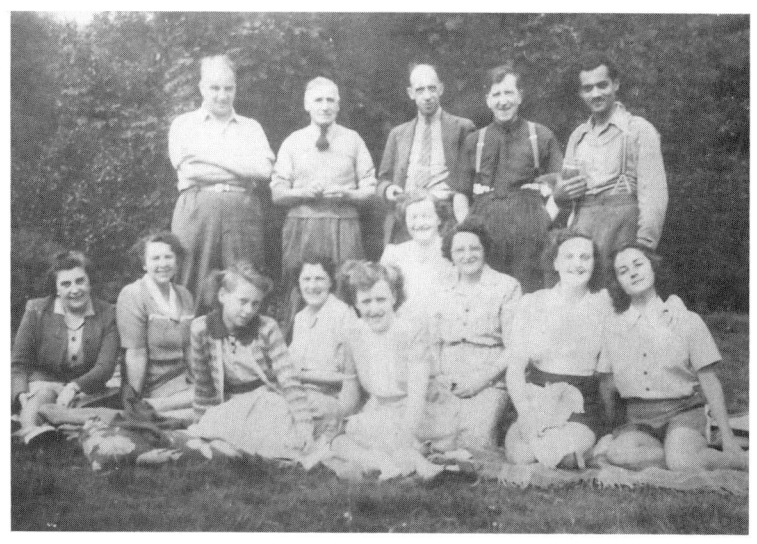

Summer picnic with Yorkshire families at Wykeham, near
Scarborough. Author at extreme right – back row.

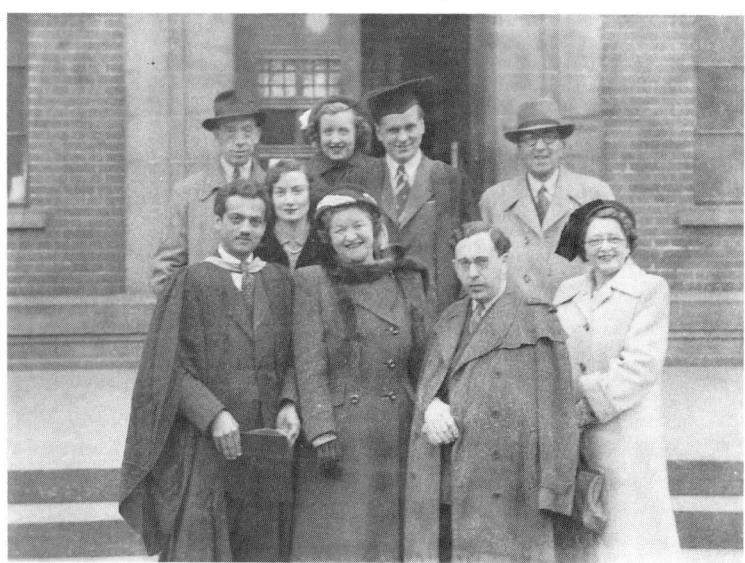

Author's 'family' at graduation, Leeds 1950. Dr Ernest
Duggleby wearing mortar board.

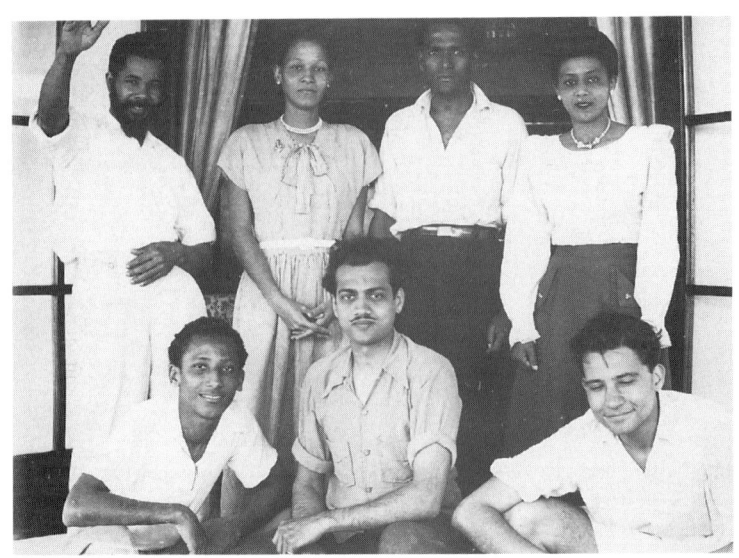

On board the "SS Matina". *Left, back row:* Uriah Butler's Lieutenant. *Front centre:* author. *Right, front row:* Dr Tony Gale.

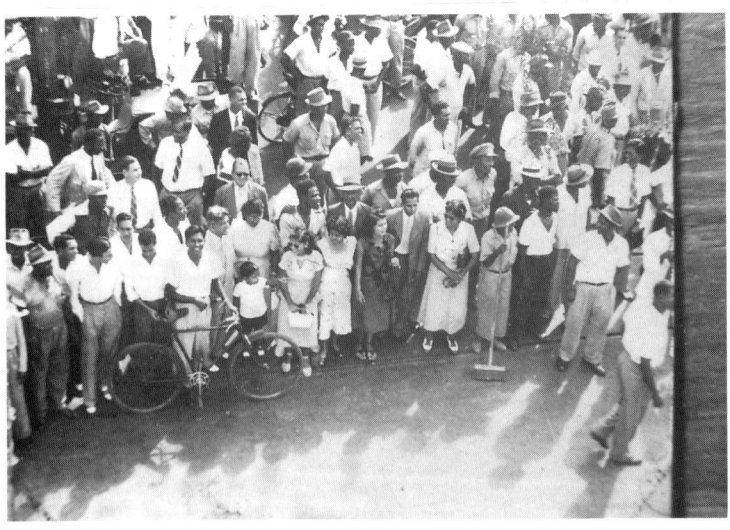

On the dock reception, Port of Spain. Author's family at centre of photograph, 1950.

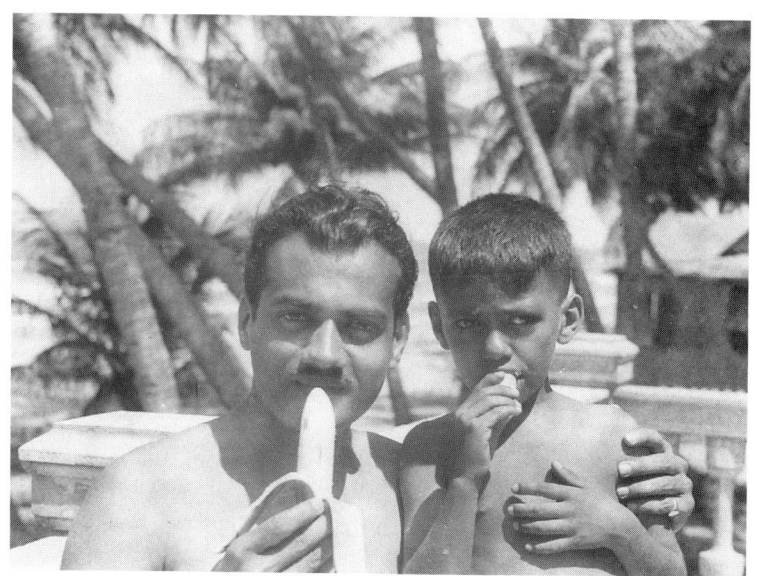

Absorbing sunshine and bananas. Author and brother
(twenty-three years apart) at Mayaro, South Trinidad East
Coast, 1950.

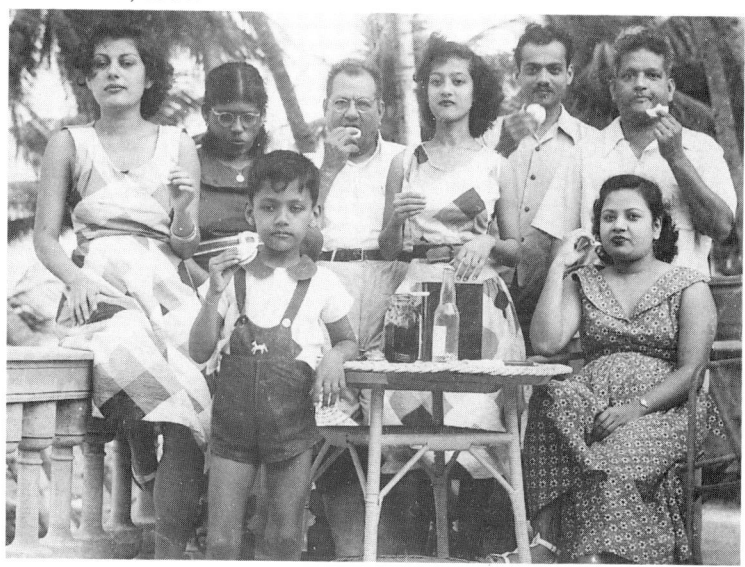

Family picnic at Mayaro, 1951.
Back row left to right: sister Annabelle, mother, father,
sister Christabelle, self, Uncle Shadrack (Chācha).
Front row left to right: brother Ronald, Aunt Dolly.

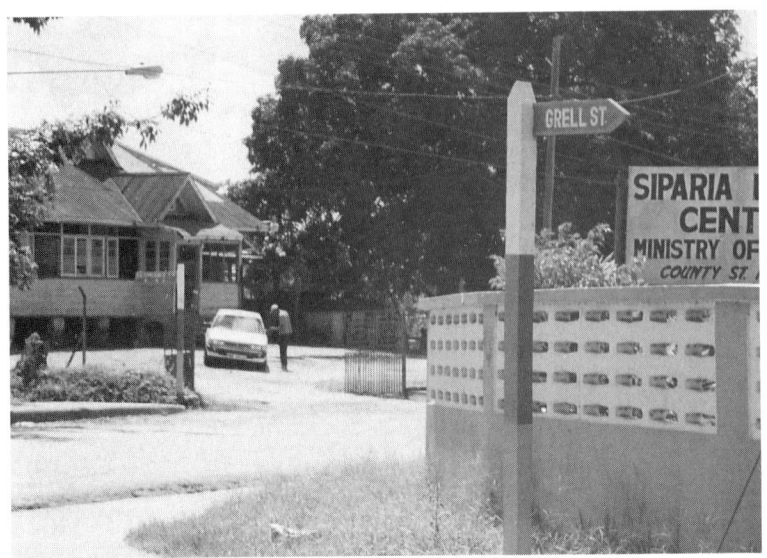

Grell Street and Old Magistrate's Quarters, 1994.

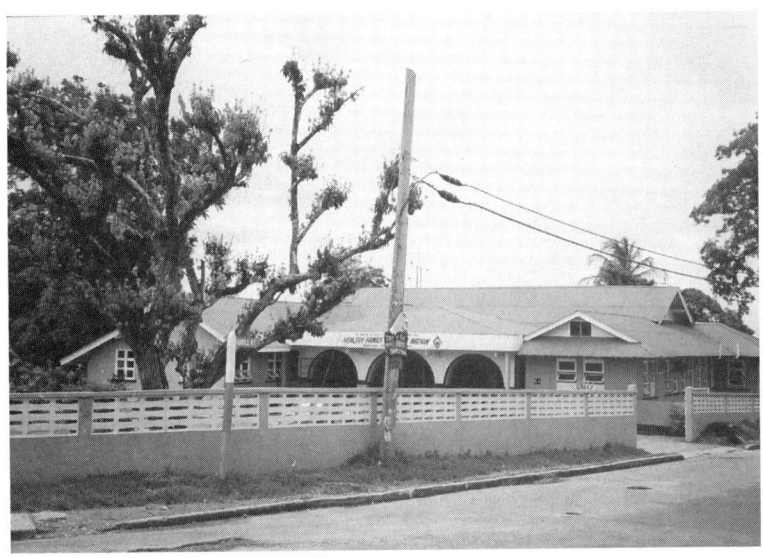

Siparia Health Centre from Grell Street, 1994.

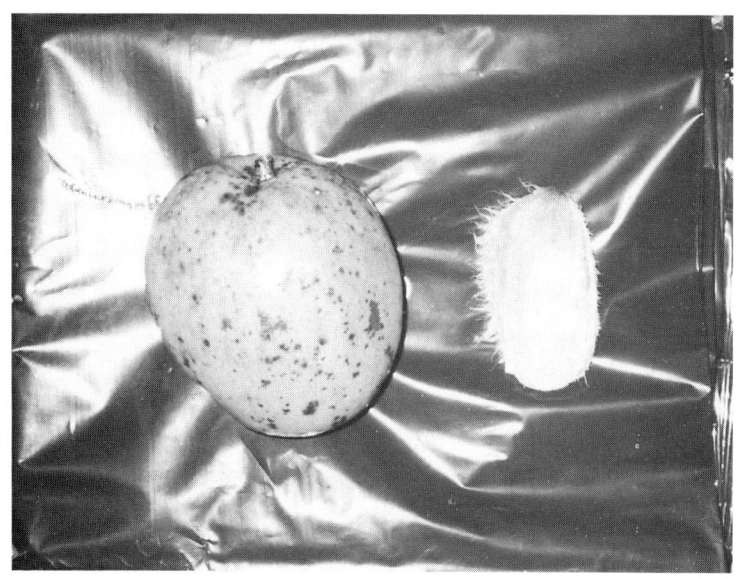

Mango variety with little fibre.

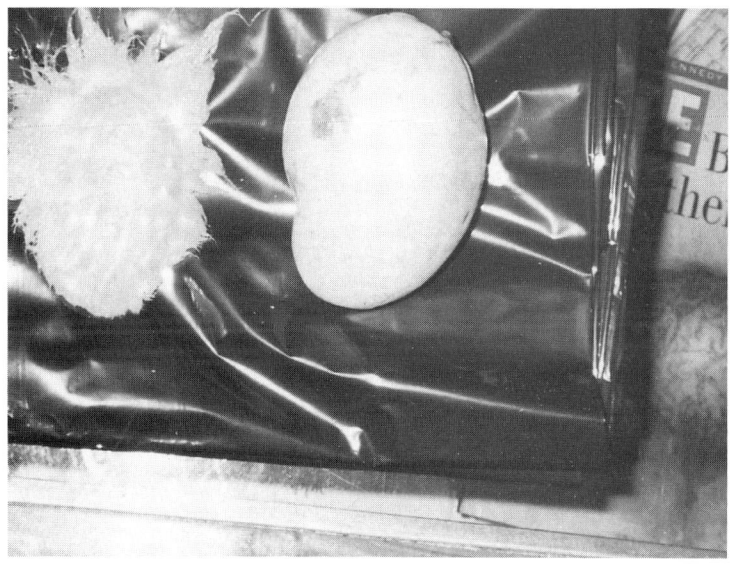

Mango variety with excessive fibre.

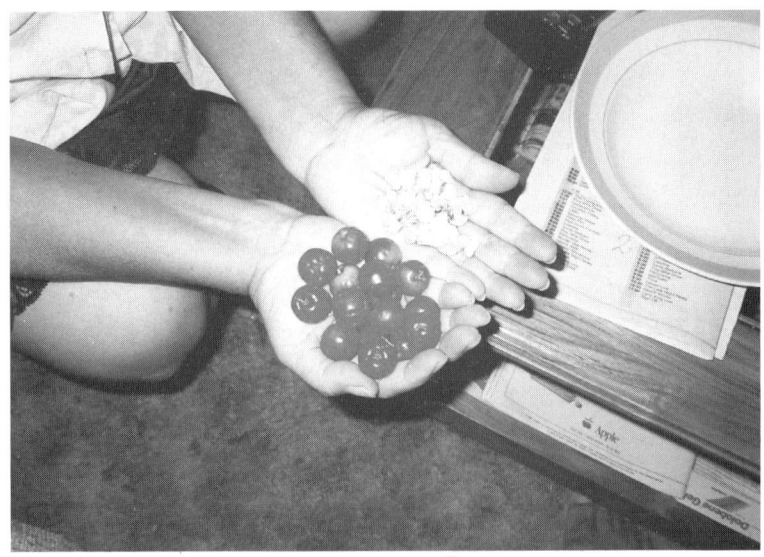

Delicious cherries and angular seeds.

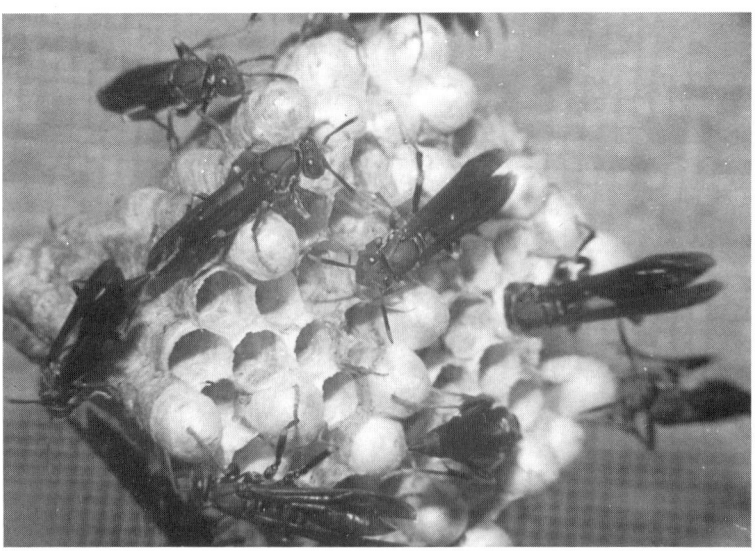

Jack Spaniard nest showing breeding cells and adults.
Photo by Dirk Sampath

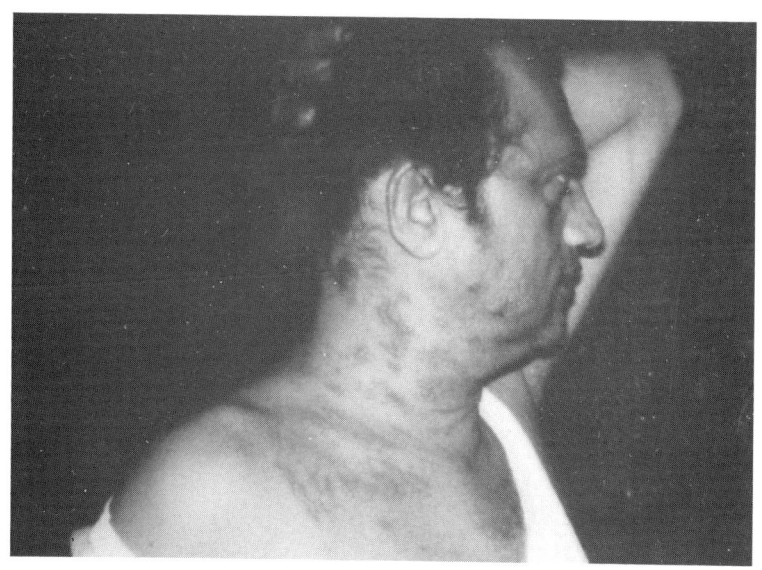

Author's shingles: Cervical 3rd nerve. Fifth day.
Photo by Cynthia Sampath

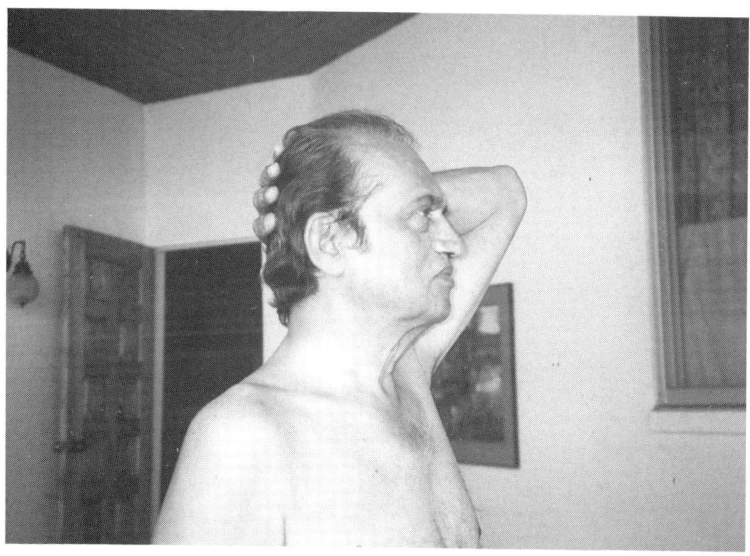

Photo by Cynthia Sampath

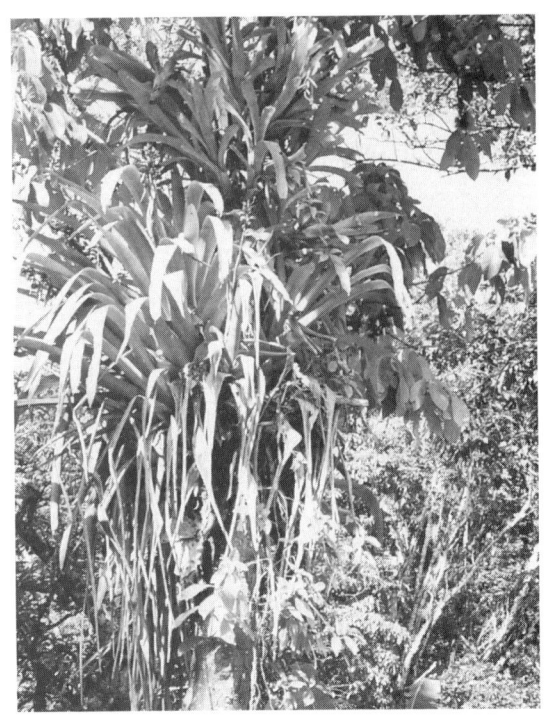

Saprophytic wild pines: breeding sites for mosquitoes.

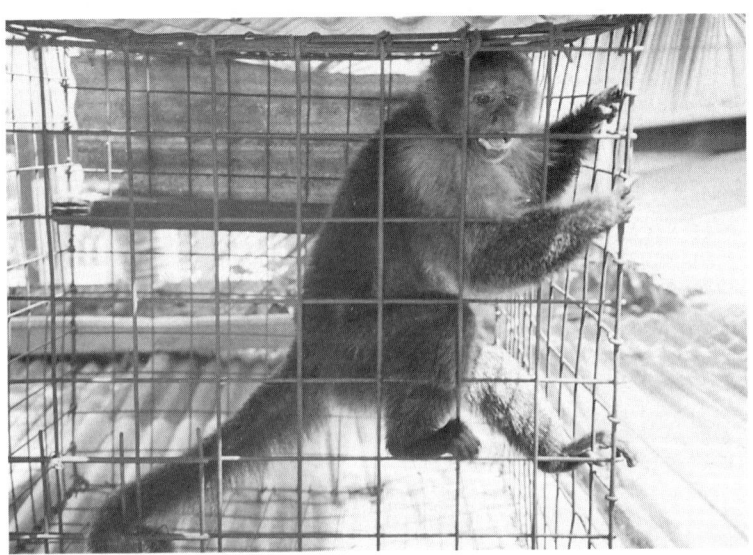

Red Howler Monkey – Yellow Fever Reservoir.

Doctors' Fees

When, as DMO, I attended to my first private patient, he asked me, "What's the damage?" I was nonplussed. I had sutured his skin-deep wound fairly neatly, and wondered whether he was concerned about residual cosmetic or functional disability. I replied that it ought to heal up perfectly if he kept it dry. "So what is the damage?" he repeated in firmer tone. "How much money?"

Only then did I realise that the word he used was the English pronunciation of the French word 'damages', which is the financial settlement in a lawsuit. On later reflection, it occurred to me that there must be something in the socio-psychology of the doctor-patient-illness relationship suggesting a contest of sorts between the doctor and the illness or injury, and the doctor having won, he was entitled to 'damages'.

Does this explanation sound too far fetched for you?

Well, read this: A person travelling by taxi will, at the end of the trip, ask the driver, "What's the damage?" and after making a purchase at the vegetable market, the housewife will ask the vendor, "What's the damage?" The explanation? Well, one must remember that in the old days – and even today in many parts of the country and of the world – bargaining for prices is the norm. The seller asks for ten dollars, the prospective purchaser offers five, the vendor says seven, the buyer offers six, the vendor demands six fifty, and the buyer agrees, so he has lost the match, and pays damages.

But what if the vendor loses the match and agrees to sell at a price lower than what it cost him? Well, then his loss is the damage he has sustained![4]

---

[4] Alternative explanations: the word 'dun' means 'to demand payment'. The word 'doomage' means 'the assessment of'. It is possible that 'damage' could be a surviving corruption of either of these almost archaic words.

The generation of doctors just before mine habitually accepted payment in kind in lieu of cash. Dr Hamilton J. Marcelin, for example, often travelled home from his Siparia office with his car trunk laden with live chickens, eggs, corn, peas, yams, cassava, bunches of bananas and so on. He was once paid with a live agouti – a wild rodent whose flesh is regarded as a delicacy by local gourmets.

When I started private practice in 1954, the standard fee for a visit ranged from $2 to $5 for an adult, and $1 to $2 for a child under twelve years of age. Generally, doctors in Port of Spain charged the higher fee, and those in the rest of the country graded the charge down. Many doctors charged the patient according to what appeared to the doctor to be the financial status of the patient. I did not think that this was right and I asked for the same fee from all. Of course, sometimes the patient would not have the full fee, and according to my mood – and perhaps some intangible other reaction – I would either write down the balance as a debt on the side of his card, or just accept whatever he paid as settlement.

I usually supplied all the medicines – at approximately cost price – so that most adults got everything for $4, and $4.50 if an injection was included, and a child paid $2 and $2.50 respectively. My competing colleague in the district, my good friend Dr Lloyd Jorsling, charged the same fees for visits as I did, but his prescriptions were filled at his father's adjoining pharmacy, so most patients paid a total of $6 or $7 for visits plus medicines. The DMOs pattern was like mine, so that many people left my friend and came to the DMO and to me. The market was too small for three doctors, and Lloyd soon left and started a very successful practice in the more affluent Port of Spain.

Even in 1954, the overall cost of medical attention was a very important factor in the choice of doctor, especially in rural areas. The international price of crude oil, which provided some 75% of our country's income, was then US$2 per barrel, and the exchange rate for our money was US$1 = TT$2.40. Gradually, the accepted fee rose to six and then to ten dollars per visit, and with the oil boom in the late 1970s, when a barrel of oil fetched US$40 in the international market, and petro-dollars, in the words of Mr Tom Adams – Prime Minister of neighbouring Barbados – were 'flowing through the economy like a dose of salts', prices of everything skyrocketed: a visit to the doctor cost $40 without medicines. In Siparia, I charged $40 for everything. Most of our medicines were imported, and, with the exchange rate moving from $2.40 to $4.25 and then to $5.90, the TT$ cost of these drugs was more than quadrupled, and even with my $40 fee, my net income fell by more than 50%, calculated in US dollars. I cannot now stock the more expensive medicines, and none of the creams and ointments, except in small quantities for use in emergencies.

During the past ten years, our economy has been in the doldrums – it has been described as 'stagflation', a paradoxical combination of stagnation and inflation. Unemployment is about 26%, food is very expensive: a pound of subsidised wheat flour (imported grain, milled locally) is $2 per pound, and subsidised sugar, fully locally grown and manufactured, is $1.50 per pound. Locally fished shrimp, most of which is exported to a thriving US market, is sold locally at $14 per pound.

The price of oil dropped to almost $10 per barrel a few years ago, and has recently risen to $17, but prices have not fluctuated in parallel with the oil income. A curious situation arose when the oil price, and hence our national income, plummeted: the shortfall was met by an *increase* in the gasoline tax, although we distil our own gasoline from our own crude oil! So that the cheaper the crude oil, the more expensive was petrol!

Most patients now go to the free health centres, and the hospital casualty departments are terribly overcrowded. Only a small percentage of patients seek private medical care – they just don't have the money after paying for their basic necessities. When in 1954 there were four, there are today fifteen doctors in the five mile radius around Siparia, and on some days we each see as few as five patients. On a busy day we may see twenty each, usually when one or two of us are ill and absent or on vacation.

On Credit

When I first started private practice, I gave a lot of 'trust', as credit is termed in Trinidad and Tobago. I soon found that I could expect eventual settlement of about 75% of these debts. People here do not budget for medical expenses, and many of these 'trust' seekers come to the private doctor for a dire emergency when the Health

Officer is unavailable, and the pain or discomfort is too great, or they do not have the money to pay the fare to the hospital fifteen miles away. Many are routine cases, seeking credit until the employed wage earner's pay day. For the first category, settlement of the debt is about 5%, and for the latter, about 70%. I do not think that most of these delinquents are dishonest. When pay day comes around they have so many other bills to pay that the doctor – who "doesn't really need the money; he have plenty already" – is left until the next pay day, by which time the patients are again broke because they have settled the bill for food, clothes, books and so on. They sometimes come for a visit months or years later, and when I point out the debt written on the card, I get varying responses, for example: "You know, ah really forget about dat," or, "But you mean to say me husband ent come to pay dat?" or, "Ah did sen' it wid me sister but like she forget," or, "I did come to pay but you did close up already," or, "I was keeping it for you but you was on holiday so long dat ah spen' it". Naturally, these delinquents have brought only enough for the current visit, and I have a stack of cards with arrows in red ink indicating the fee which the patient had incurred at a previous visit !

But some are downright dishonest: a woman came in one day with a card recording previous visits, but the card was a few millimetres narrower than the standard. I called this to the receptionist's attention and she smilingly told me that there had been a balance of $5 entered on the card. The clever lady had performed a neat surgical liquidation of her debt!

A young lady brought her seven month old infant to see me. Her face looked familiar, and I asked her whether I had attended to her before.

"Oh yes," she replied, "When I was at school you sewed up a cut on my foot." My receptionist looked up the old files and found her card. Seven years before, I had, indeed, sutured a deep axe wound on the dorsum of her right foot, and her mother had no money at all so I wrote down a balance of $7 on her card, and her mother promised to settle when she returned to get the sutures out in seven days time.

"Didn't you come back to remove the stitches?" I asked.

"Oh", she replied, "Mummy took me to the Health Office to take them out."

Several debt entries have been erased in my waiting room by finger and spittle!

But there are some very conscientious people. One afternoon in the 1960s, as I was about to leave the office, a young woman, of about twenty-five, came in, obviously in labour. I found that she was almost fully dilated. It was her second delivery, and her pains were strong. She would certainly have given birth on her way to hospital, on the pot-holed fifteen mile road, with the rush of on-coming homeward bound traffic of four in the afternoon. She delivered uneventfully, placenta and all, within fifteen minutes. I gave her the required shot of ergometrine, and cleaned her and the baby up, wrapped him up, and asked my receptionist to get a taxi for her. She had no money except the taxi fare, and I wrote down a balance of $20 on her card.

She came in again one year later, in exactly the same circumstances as to time, diagnosis and prognosis, but with one difference: on this occasion, she was accompanied by a young man, the reputed father of the arriving infant. While I was examining the expectant mother, my receptionist again smilingly brought in her card (she was quite used to this situation) with the old balance written on it. Everything came through quite normally, and when the father asked the fee, I told him twenty dollars, and pointed out that the lady still owed me for her previous delivery. He replied that he had only thirty dollars, and although the elder infant had another father, he would pay the remainder of the outstanding bill as well when he got some more money. He paid thirty dollars there and then, and one week later he returned and paid the ten dollars as promised.

One midnight in 1952, I was awakened at the DMOs quarters, and asked to visit a woman who had delivered, but whose afterbirth had been retained for several hours. After stopping the car about four miles away, I was conducted along a muddy trace by flashlight for about a mile until we arrived at an ajoupa in which, by flambeau (a bottle filled with kerosene and a lighted wick at the opening), I saw a young, exhausted perspiring woman lying with a tiny infant between her legs, still attached by its umbilical cord to its mother. She was bleeding. I gave an injection of pitocin, plus ergometrine, ligated and separated the cord, and asked that she be given sugar water to drink, as much as she wanted. The placenta came out whole, and immediately a tiny head appeared. I delivered the twin infant, and laid him alongside his brother. The second placenta was delivered easily, and the bleeding stopped. All three patients, despite their ordeal, looked quite strong, and I asked the father to let me see all of them after three days at my office. He asked me what my fee was, and I told him seven dollars. They were obviously very poor, and I felt that a token sum would be appropriate for preserving both his and my self-esteem.

I noticed that the father was a very heavy smoker – he finished at least three cigarettes during my visit – and that the babies, albeit twins, were very small. At that time, I did not know the connection between passive nicotine inhalation and birth weight.

They never came to my office and for forty-two years I agonised over their apparent ingratitude. How could anyone act thus, after all the trouble to which I had been put, after I had saved three lives, and charged merely a small token fee? I was not angry. It was a gnawing, hollow sadness, akin to the pangs of unrequited love.

On Tuesday 14th June, 1994, a woman of about fifty-two came to visit me, and after the consultation, as she was about to leave, the following conversation ensued.

"Doctor, you do not remember me, but I remember you very well."

"Did I attend to you when you were a child?"

"No, but you attended to my mother at our house."

"What complaint did your mother have?"

"She couldn't make her babies, and you delivered them."

"Where did you live?"

"In a trace, off the Guapo Road to Fyzabad."

I immediately remembered the occasion – and the debt.

"How are they getting on?"

"Oh, Ma did all right, but the babies died."

"How did they die?"

"Well, the first one lived for a month, but the second one lasted only a week. My father took them to jharray, but they never caught themselves. We were very poor, there were six of us, and my mother did not have enough breast milk, and the babies did not strive on the condensed milk and flour pap she was giving them."

So it was not ingratitude after all: it was the stark constraint of abject poverty. I was sorry that the infants did not survive after all that we went through, but the burden of sadness which I had nursed for four decades lifted completely from my mind.

A National Health Plan

Since the early 1950s, I had been convinced that for primary health care, this country needed a prepaid health plan, so that sick persons could get early medical attention, without having to pay at the time of the visit. My experience with life threatening situations, which could have been avoided if early medical attention had been sought, and which was not sought because of the absence of cash, convinced me even further of this need. My difficulties with credit merely underlined this sentiment.

My recommendation, that a small sub-committee be appointed by the Trinidad and Tobago Medical Association to produce a skeleton form of proposal in connection with this, resulted in the following which was published in the Caribbean Medical Journal Vol. 35 (1&2) of 1974.

TTMA Proposals for a Prepaid Voluntary Health Plan for Trinidad and Tobago

Sub-Committee: Drs Sampath, Jorsling, Gunness, Gaskin

Ultimate Aim: A full comprehensive prepaid health plan.

Definitions: *Full comprehensive*: To embrace all members of the population.
Pre-paid: No payment for service or treatment, including drugs at the time of medical attention. All payments to be made regularly in advance, whether the member is healthy or ill.

Agency: A National Health Corporation.

Authority: A statutory board.

Revenue Sources:
(a) Compulsory deductions from the wages of wage earners.

(b) Optional monthly contributions from self employed persons. Those who do not join the plan will not be eligible for attention under the plan.

(c) Contributions from Government based on a sum (to be fixed) for each person recommended by their agency as being unemployed or unemployable. (In general terms this will cover poor persons, paupers, pensioners, medically disabled persons etc.)

Recommendation of these persons will be the task of government, presumably through their pensions and poor relief agencies. The corporation will issue membership cards to these persons, and they will be entitled to full medical care. There will be no 'second class' members.

All monies from the above sources, will be pooled in a 'Health Insurance Fund', to be administered by the 'National Health Corporation'.

All lands, buildings equipment etc., now controlled by the Ministry of Health, in particular hospitals, health offices etc., to be transferred to the National Health Corporation.

All private hospitals, industrial medical facilities, private medical practitioners will be permitted to function outside the plan, if they wish, and all private insurance companies will be permitted to function, if they desire.

All industrial concerns will be invited to donate their facilities to the corporation, which will undertake to treat their employees as part of the comprehensive plan.

All medical practitioners will be invited to join the plan, and to be paid according to a schedule on a per capita list basis, plus a fee for service basis, or some modification thereof, to be decided by members of the Medical Association themselves.

Salaries at hospitals, including out-patients, to be fixed by the Board. It is anticipated that many of the more simple surgical procedures will be done by private practitioners (as a result of cost of service payment), so that the casualty load will be lightened. Surgeons, including assistants, will be paid (in addition to monthly salaries) a fee per operation.

STAFFING:

HOSPITALS:

It is anticipated that the increased emoluments and incentives offered will result in more than a full complement, so that extra leisure for rest and study will be available to staff, which in itself will be an incentive. Private practitioners will be encouraged to participate in hospital work. Questions of study leave etc. are to be worked out in detail.

CENTRES OUTSIDE HOSPITALS:

Apart from an eight hour daytime service on week days supplied by private practitioners, a sixteen-hour, six days per week service, plus a twenty-four Sunday service, will be supplied at specified district hospitals and health centres throughout the islands. This service will be manned by private practitioners on a rota system, and payment will be at a rate approximately one and a half times those for normal working hours.

DENTAL SERVICE

We recommend that the Dental Association be invited to consider whether they will desire to participate. If they do, then their proposals could be incorporated. If they do not, then for the moment, dental care will not be included in the plan.

SCHEDULE OF COST PER SERVICE PAYMENTS TO DOCTORS:

To be based on the insurance plans already in existence, but will be somewhat less. This will not be a disadvantage because the volume of service will be far greater. We should consider suggesting to Government, that doctors could, by way of "pioneer" activity, ask for a fraction of the costs stipulated by the present insurance companies, and be exempted from income tax.

SPECIAL SERVICES:

For example, to insurance companies (life policies), embassies for immigration, private companies (examination for fitness), police examinations and so on, to be included in the schedule. To pay directly to doctor, as private service, or to pay to the Corporation which will then pay to the doctor.

*

The desirability of a National Health Plan had been the subject of discussion at least since the 1940s. Dr J.A. Waterman, the founder and first editor of the Caribbean Medical Journal, and sometime Acting Director of Medical Services, was a proponent of a modified 'Blue Cross' plan, and the Medical Association had discussed the formulation of other plans, from the 1950s onwards. One such discussion was led by Dr Winston Mahabir, before he became Minister of Health. In October 1966, a seventy-two page comprehensive document was laid before the Cabinet by Ms Isabel U. Teshea, Minister of Health, and was approved by that Cabinet eleven years later on 27th June, 1977. We at the TTMA flattered ourselves that it was our prodding which stimulated this result. But still no plan has been put into operation!

Always before the medical and lay public are the problems of the British scheme, the Canadian plan, and now the difficulties and criticisms of President Clinton's efforts in the USA. We now have quite a formidable government plan before us in Trinidad and Tobago, but the criticisms continue. Will we ever have in operation a truly National Health Scheme?

By Any Other Name

Ninety percent of patients know their own, and their children's, names and surnames and maiden names when applicable, but the remaining ten percent are a source of repeated search and research on the part of my receptionists.

A knowledge of the social and familial backgrounds in our country is necessary in order to understand why this is so.

Among persons of East Indian ethnicity, surnames were originally not used, and occasionally only caste names, for example, Maharaj or Singh, were used as surnames. As these older heads had children, the father's given name was used as a surname. But the first name of the child is not always consistently used, so that a child may be called by one name as an infant, another in babyhood, a third in early childhood, and another as an adult. This is sometimes complicated by the fact that occasionally the grandfather's name is given as the child's surname, especially when the child is brought to the doctor by the grandmother. Very often, the relative escorting the child knows him, or her, only by a pet name, such as 'baby', 'girlsin', 'boboy', 'chunks' and so on.

There have been numerous instances of same name and surname. Among my cards, there is a very striking occurrence of two 'Dolly Soodoosingh's', who lived at Penal Rock Road and Penal Pluck Road respectively. They were completely unrelated, and strangers to each other, but were the same age, got married at about the same time and had their pregnancies and deliveries almost coincidentally. They were very different in appearance, but for many years they came in from the waiting room with each other's card given to them in error. I discovered the mix-up only when I was doing a survey of distribution of pigmentation in the general population, as a baseline for comparison with the distribution of employees in banks, when I was a member of a Government Commission charged with investigating race and colour discrimination in employment in banks. I used colour photographs of persons, ranging in colour from white to black on a scale of one to six, and wrote the appropriate number on each patient's card. One Dolly was three on the scale, and the other was five. When one Dolly came in with the other's card, the number did not match, and I pointed this out to my receptionist, and underlined in red the words 'Rock' and 'Pluck'. We never confused them after this. There are very many persons with the same names, but it is usually easy to give the right cards by looking at the age and the address. But there are at least three of my patients who have name, age and address exactly the same, and, indeed, they are of approximately the same colour! They can be distinguished only by checking the date of their last visit, and confirming by questioning, what was the nature of the ailment.

Among persons of African descent, the name problem arises very often as a result of the extremely prevalent common law relationships. Surnames may be that of the mother, of the biological father, or of the second head of the household. The mother has difficulty in remembering what surname was given on each occasion. I have had as many as four different cards with four different surnames for the same patient.

On a very few occasions, my alert receptionist remembers what name was given before, and, on finding the correct card, she sometimes finds that a small balance is entered on that card!

I should not want readers to conclude that difficulty with payment of fees and with names, and the dishonesty rarely associated with them, are a formidable problem. They are not, and are recounted here only because the challenge and the humour that these instances introduce into what would otherwise be a routine – even humdrum practice (and narrative) – deserve to be shared, if only vicariously, with my non-medical and medical colleagues.

Shy Patients and Children

Wednesday 21st December, 1994: This morning, a young man of twenty, well-dressed and softly spoken, came in to see me, and asked for "something for a rash".

"Where do you have the rash?" I enquired.

"Down below here," he replied indicating his crotch.

"On your thighs, or on your penis?"

"On the penis."

"Well, let me have a look."

"Oh it scratches and has little sores on it."

"Okay Let me see what it looks like."

"Do you really have to see it?"

"Of course. If I don't examine it, I will be treating you by guess work, and may not give you the correct treatment."

"Can't you tell what it is by my description?"

"No, I can't. Don't be shy, I have seen thousands of these things, but I cannot treat them unless I examine them."

"I cannot let you see it." And he left.

This has been my first experience of a patient refusing to let me see his or her genital area! Virginal ladies are often shy, but their timidity usually never exceeds a transient reluctance to part their thighs, but a very common occurrence is the following.

A woman – and she may be quite mature with several children – complains of anything: headaches, dizzy spells, tiredness and so on, and after a thorough examination, including visual acuity, blood pressure, heart, lungs, reflexes, urine specimen and so on, I may find only a slight anaemia, and prescribe iron and vitamins. She pays her fee, and as she approaches the door, she turns and says, "Oh doctor, I nearly forgot to tell you. I have a discharge (or an itching) down below."

She is a shy person, and this complaint is what she really came to see me about, but was able to summon up sufficient courage to tell me only at the very last minute. Sometimes, I wonder whether I should ask all persons with vague symptoms and no obvious signs, the leading question about their genital areas, and so save some of them the embarrassment of having to volunteer such complaint.

Many years ago, a young, pregnant bride was brought to me by her mother-in-law, and was very reluctant to let me examine her vaginally. The older lady said to her, "Girl, don't be stupid eh! The doctor see bellyful already!" What she meant, by this common Trinidadian expression, was that the doctor was satiated with such examinations, and that he took only a professional interest in the procedure.

As it happened, the mother-in-law was suffering from cirrhosis of the liver, and much later I called once a month at their home to tap the fluid from her abdomen. By this time, the young bride was her constant nurse and helper, and already had two daughters aged nine and seven. When I withdrew the needle and rubber tubing, these children eagerly assisted in washing them out with soap and water. Later, when these girls had their first pregnancies, their mother brought them to me, and she recounted to them her own first experience with my medical attention. They were never shy, and I am looking forward to providing a grandfather figure image for *their* girls in similar circumstances.

Many babies and young children are afraid of the doctor. In most instances, they have received their 'shots' against infectious diseases, and it is an anticipatory fear of the needle. In other instances, it is a fear inculcated by the parent, who has threatened the child that if he or she does not stop sucking his or her finger, the doctor will cut it off. Sometimes, the threat is to cut off the tongue, so that the doctor is well advised to discard his metal spatula – which the child may interpret to be a knife – and use a disposable wooden tongue depressor for the absolutely vital examination of a child's throat.

I always appreciate it when parents bringing a child for the first time, also bring an accompanying older sibling who has been a veteran patient of mine, with whom I can chat and pretend to examine, so as to demonstrate to the younger child that I am a harmless old friend of the family. I have often heard a child of three or four tell a fearful, weeping younger brother or sister that the doctor is 'nice' and 'wouldn't do you anything!'

I have seen my third generation of children. Will I enjoy the privilege of seeing a fourth?

Anatomical Concepts

Many people do not know the names of their body parts. One will complain of a pain in his 'stomach', and point to his chest. The word 'foot' is universally used to denote the entire limb, from groin to the tip of the toes, and the 'hand', correspondingly, refers collectively to everything from the shoulders to the fingers. One hears references to the 'fingers' and 'palms' of the feet. I suspect that the term 'sole', having the same pronunciation as 'soul', is, in our religious society, regarded as somewhat blasphemous if applied to the lowest level of the body.

But anatomical misnaming is not the exclusive province of the unlearned or unsophisticated. On one occasion, while giving evidence in court, I described to the jury in a murder case (which after my evidence, was relegated to manslaughter) an injury, one inch wide through the front of the chest, which had penetrated the victim's heart. It had cut through the cartilage of the inner ends of a rib on its journey inwards. I had seen the instrument – a very sharp and pointed brushing cutlass – at the scene of the incident (a rum shop on the Siparia Road) and when asked in court what degree of force was used, I replied, "Moderate force". The learned judge appeared surprised that moderate force would be sufficient to produce such dire consequences, and he asked me, "Would it not be necessary to use very great force to penetrate such a bony *diaphragm*?" I realised immediately that my reply would have to be given with the most tactful choice of words: "My Lord," I replied, with measured deference in my tone of voice, "that part of the body is usually called by us doctors the 'rib cage', and the instrument in this case just happened – quite by unlucky chance – to make contact with the soft cartilage which joins the bony rib to the hard breast bone; if it had touched a mere one and a half inches on either side, it would have met bone and would not have penetrated the chest cavity. Incidentally, my

Lord, we doctors refer to the soft internal muscle barrier between the chest and the abdomen as the *diaphragm.*"

Even a reputable and otherwise erudite magazine such as *Time* can have an anatomical lapse: on page twenty-four of its August 17th, 1992 international issue, for example, the opening paragraph read, 'With his crazy stare, massive knuckles and tattooed *biceps*, Jimmy T. looks like an urban...' The accompanying photograph showed a subject with a huge tattoo, depicting a man with a gun, on his *deltoid*, and nothing on his biceps.

Despite my mailed correction, no mention was made of the error in any subsequent issue of this prestigious magazine, and millions of young Americans and others now have an authorising precedent for this anatomical misconception.

The 'Little Fellow' and Other Sobriquets

A man of fifty, a regular patient of mine, father of six children, all of them my patients, the youngest being eleven months old, had a sore throat which I treated. As he was about to leave he said to me:

"Doctor, the little fellow has trouble standing up."

"If you hold him, does he stand up?"

"A little bit, but he falls down when I let him go."

"Well it's not unusual at that age. Let me check him out some time."

"What about now?" replied he, indicating his crotch.

The word 'penis' is derived from the Latin for 'tail', something hanging down, a pendant as it were. British polite society, after Julius Caesar, the Roman conquerors and, presumably, their new middle class collaborators among the conquered Britons, must have forsworn the use of the more expressive and militant sounding 'cock'. This word and its functionally expressive companion 'prick' are commonly used in Trinidad and Tobago. In our own polite society, these words are regarded as too 'common', suitable, as in ancient Britain only, for use by the plebeians. Another synonym is 'tool' – a functional word – and several polite variations are current in Trinbago, for example, 'Tor', 'Toto', 'Totee', 'Toteelo' and 'Torcas'.

'Coco' appears to be a polite variation of 'Cock', but 'John Thomas', 'Johnny Boy', 'John Holmes', and 'Golden Boy' do not immediately suggest their derivations or implications, except perhaps to indicate that this organ sometimes appears to possess an individuality and personality of its own, beyond the control of its owner.

As a cricketing nation, the expressive, functional synonym 'willow' – the 'wood' (also a synonym) of the cricket bat – is much employed, and has given rise to its diminutive 'willie'.

Its fancied resemblance to the bird of that name, has suggested 'pigeon' and 'pidgee' for short. The names 'sword' and 'bolo' (after the bolo knife?) are used, possibly in deference to its propensity for cleavage. Diminutives sometimes used are 'boles' and 'bolsee'.

The terms 'lolo', 'lollie', 'wiggie' and 'kickilee' appear to be a type of visual onomatopoeia for the flaccid state; 'lollipop', however may be used in deference to the propensity of the 'lolo' occasionally to attain erectility.

A well-educated radio announcer who is highly respected and very respectable and religious with a well-developed social conscience – she was at one time selected to meet the Pope and to kiss his ring – wrote to one of our daily newspapers deploring the obscene contortions of some of our female masqueraders. She particularly objected to their 'showing their vaginas' during their winding on the streets during Carnival. One correspondent replied in print, correcting her anatomical inaccuracy. It was impossible, he noted, for the organ she had named to be visible or even outlined, no matter what posture was adopted by the young ladies she criticised. She had named a sequestered part to include the whole! Indeed, her criticism could have been more properly directed to one of our salacious weekly newspapers which makes a point of publishing photographs of our young ladies in which this anatomical area is clearly and usually exaggeratedly outlined on almost every page.

The dear lady correspondent obviously had very good moral intentions but should have said 'pudenda', however, this word is not known to many. Even the word 'vulva' would not have been accurate, since, technically, it refers only to the oval shaped orifice and does not include the labia and the pubis which are the eye-catching focus of the onlooker.

My patients have a variety of names for this area and its constituent parts: As with the male counterpart, the Anglo-Saxon word 'cunt' and its derivative 'cunnie', have become obscene swearwords and are never heard in my respectable office. My patients refer zoologically to 'cat', 'pussy', 'pussy-cat', 'butterfly' and 'salt fish'. In Hindi, that part is referred to as the 'boor', or in English, 'bear'. A common Hindi cussing phrase is *'Tohar mai ki boor'*, which means 'Your mother's bear'. Then there are numerous terms of endearment, examples are, 'pat-a-cake', 'rosie', 'pinkie', 'tun-tun', 'toonie', 'coon-coon' – possibly a euphemism for the cruder 'cunt' – 'poky' and 'kitty' – obviously a small cat. It is sometimes referred to as the 'old lady', and 'nani', the Hindi for one's maternal grandmother. A recent calypso which described how a taxi driver, 'lick up me nani', was condemned for weeks in the local press for its apparent *double entendre*.

The Influenzas

Epidemics of influenza or 'the flu' invade us each year. It enters regularly at Port of Spain and our airport at Piarco, and within days or weeks spreads southward. Then, within a month to six weeks, having wrought its havoc in varying degrees, it finally disappears until another strain enters our population the following year. Patients are suddenly, unexpectedly, and often completely knocked out and can be bed-ridden for five days. In Trinidad and Tobago, with our innate propensity for picturesque synonyms, we have not allowed our influenzas to escape – perhaps as a psychological shield. If you can identify your enemy by name, he is at once less mysterious, more tangible, even more frangible!

When the Asian flu first hit us in the 1950s, we called it by the name given to us. Another year we called it 'Jaws', after the great white shark of movie fame. One year, a woman charged with the vicious murder of her husband was acquitted. The contemporaneous flu epidemic was promptly named 'Jaitoon' in her honour. We also christened our invaders 'Kung Fu', 'Wang You' and 'Rambo' after their simultaneous macho appearance on our movie screens. 'Skylab' soon followed as that space station came hurtling down unchecked, and the year the government introduced some stringent fiscal measures, its flu was trinologically named 'Budget'. Other influenza epidemics were named, 'Abu Bakr', after a man who led an unsuccessful, violent political coup, and 'Gilbert', the hurricane which devastated much of the Greater Antilles. Late 1994 additions were 'Hijab', named after a violent controversy regarding this Islamic attire worn by a schoolgirl, 'The Sting', after a police operation, and in 1995, 'Buckle-up', when seatbelts became mandatory.

Cancer

I have found that patients with cancer need to be told frankly about their ailment and what to expect. Nowadays the prospects are excellent when diagnosed early, and several of my patients have had complete cures. There are two which have stuck in my mind and which I use as examples in order to encourage others similarly afflicted.

One woman of fifty developed breast cancer. She had a radical mastectomy followed by radiotherapy. She lived to be ninety-five.

Another with cancer of the uterus, which I diagnosed when she was sixty-five, took her radiotherapy and chemotherapy – her tumour had spread extensively but locally. She is now eighty and in excellent health and always, when I meet her socially, she is obviously very happy and enjoying life almost to the full.

But there are those, some of them quite young – thirty to forty – in whom the disease has spread to the stage of inoperability. Radiotherapy and chemotherapy have not arrested the condition, and some of them suffer constant, severe pain, only praying for death to end their travail. Unlike Dr Kevorkian, I do not believe in assisting their departure. Perhaps if I, or a very close relative, were in that condition, I might change my attitude. I really do not know.

I give the relatives of such sufferers adequate amounts of Sosegon tablets, at the wholesale cost price, to be used liberally whenever necessary and as often as necessary. Both patient and relatives are extremely grateful for the assistance of this powerful painkiller which I now supply only for these cases.

Spoons, Tablets and Millilitres

Very often when I give a mother enough liquid medicine for four days because I need and wish to note the child's progress at that time, she returns on the appointed day with the bottle still half full. "Have you been giving the child the medicines as written on the label: 'One teaspoonful three times per day?'"

"Oh yes, I never missed a dose."

She is telling the truth, but when I show her a 5 ml teaspoon, she remarks, "My spoon is smaller than that."

In the old days, before antibiotics, it didn't matter much how accurate the spoon was. If a cough syrup, antacid or most other remedies were slightly over or underdosed, the patient's reaction would be minimally different to what was expected. All throughout my practice, the transition to metric has remained dormant and confusing to patients. One mother, for whose baby I prescribed 5 ml, was actually using a calibrated dropper, and giving 0.5 ml at a time. I have now got into the habit of ensuring that the parent understands that a 'teaspoon' is 5 ml, and enquire whether he or she has one of the calibrated cups often supplied with non-prescription medicines. If they do not have one, I either give them one or write them a note to the nearest pharmacy to get one.

There is no problem with tablets since they are accurately manufactured in milligrams. Sometimes when prescribing for a child four years old – and sometimes up to nine years old – the mother complains, "But this child can't swallow tablets!" Now the cost of a 125 mg dose, half a tablet of 250 mg, may be 25 cents, while the cost of the equivalent in a liquid suspension may be up to four times that price. For a rich person who does not mind paying $15 for a bottle of antibiotic, it does not matter, but for a poor person, $4 for an equivalent eight tablets, the saving is substantial. I therefore encourage mothers to get their children to swallow tablets, even pieces at a time. Even for babies, the correct dose crushed in sugar water or condensed milk (available in 90% of households) is much more accurate than a 'teaspoon' of the manufactured syrup.

One trick which I often recommend is to stick the tablet into a small piece of banana which enables it to go slitheringly down the hatch.

Identical Twins

Babies who develop from the same fertilised egg (monozygotic) are, as is well known, similar both physically and mentally. I have attended to eight pairs of identical twins in the course of my practice, and I enter on their record cards some of their minor differences so that I can identify them correctly when I see them again.

My first contact with a pair of these occurred before I became a doctor: it was at a birthday party that I saw these two lovely eighteen year old ladies. They were dressed alike, and I could not tell one from the other by looking at them or by listening to their voices. But, when I danced with each of them in turn I found that one of them was decidedly lighter on her feet, and responded to my lead with greater precision and alacrity. Since then, I have always been intrigued by minor differences in so-called identical twins.

Some of these differences are: moles in different places, different shades in pigmentation, presence of a broader thumb, a capillary haemangioma (birthmark) on only one of them, and birth weight differences, the rule due undoubtedly to uterine placing and a varied placental or umbilical blood flow. The lighter twin usually catches up within a few months, but the other differences are permanent.

They have the same level of intelligence, judging by their performance at school, but there is usually a striking difference in their personalities, a difference discernible very early by their parents and associates and even by the doctor during the limited duration of their visits to him. One twin is usually more extrovert and adventurous, takes more chances, runs more risks, while the other tends to be more cautious, acting often as the conscience of the other, almost as if in the division of their common zygote they received complementary rather than identical psyches.

One mother told me that whenever one of her twin girls started to do anything dangerous, like climbing a ladder, the other would hold the base of the ladder and warn her sister to be careful!

One day, while driving slowly through California (a village north of San Fernando, Trinidad), I spied two little girls who appeared to be identical playing in their yard. I stopped and looked closely at them: they were identical. I asked their mother's permission to photograph them and she complied.

"What are their names?" I enquired.

"Annabelle and Christabelle," she told me, to my very great astonishment.

"Where did you get those lovely names from?"

"Well, my sister who lives at Penal Rock Road, visited me soon after the twins were born, and told me that she knew two pretty girls in her district with those names, and I liked the names too."

"Do you know," I told the mother, "I know those two girls very well. They are my sisters, and if you had triplets you might have named the third one after my other sister, Rosabelle!"

Acu-Points

One day in the 1960s, a middle-aged Chinese woman came to see me. She spoke no English, and unhappily I speak no Chinese. She pointed to a spot on her left big toe, then to the hypodermic needles on my desk. She obviously wanted me to inject her big toe at the spot she indicated. I examined the toe minutely, there was nothing wrong with it. I shrugged my shoulders and shook my head, trying to indicate to her that there was no need for an injection. She insisted and actually took up a needle and handed it to me and pointed to the desired spot again. 1 did not know what to make of it, so to humour her I sterilised the spot, inserted the needle, and, as I was about to withdraw it, she held my hand and walked into the side room, with the needle in situ.

I attended to three more patients – about half an hour – before she walked in again and motioned for me to withdraw the needle. She handed me a dollar, and when I refused to take it, she dropped it on my desk and left.

She returned one week later and pointed to a spot slightly higher up the foot actually at the junction between the big toe and the foot – the metatarso-phalangeal joint. She made me repeat the dry injection again for another dollar, and so, week after week, she returned for nine more weeks, each time receiving her dry injection a little higher up; ankle, leg, inner side of the thigh. At this stage, I began to wonder how high up she wanted me to go, but she never returned.

I felt very guilty for accepting her money for these innocent procedures until I read about acupuncture. In 1982, I visited a book store in Beijing and bought a book entitled, *The way to locate acu-points*, edited by Professor Yang Jiasan and translated into English by Drs Meng Xiankun and Li Xuewe. On page fifty-two, I discovered that I had unwittingly administered acupuncture to the dear lady on one of her Yin channels – the Spleen Channel of Foot Taivin!

I often wondered whether she had a malarial spleen? And did my ignorant punctures do her any good?

Albinism[5]

The absence of pigment can occur as a rarity in all animal species. In the wild, the chances of survival of an albino animal are poor: they are conspicuous targets for their predators, and tragically the same is psychologically true in the human jungle.

In my practice I have met three albino persons, two of East Indian and one of African genetic origin. George has an albino sister and a normally pigmented brother. His parents are pigmented and cannot recall any albinos in their ancestry. George is well above average in intelligence, has always taken adequate precautions against the sun, and uses polaroid glasses to protect his eyes. In his professional work, he is a competent computer operator. He is happily married to a charming, normally pigmented lady. (I had the honour of giving a speech on her behalf at their wedding!)

Andersen has normally pigmented parents and a normally pigmented sister. He is well protected from the sun, wears dark shades, and is doing very well in school. Like George, he must get close to his text for reading and prefers large type. There are no known albinos in his ancestry.

Blanco, unfortunately, is not so well endowed intellectually, socially or economically. As DMO, I detected an early epithelioma on his forearm which was successfully excised. He is now forty years old, and as a garbage collector he is constantly exposed to the merciless sun with the sparsest of protection for his eyes and skin.

My enquiries do not reveal any common ancestors for these three persons.

---

[5] It is thought that albinism is inherited as recessive genes – so called 'homozygous epistatic allelomorphs' – which are distinct from the regular genes for pigmentation.

Cremations

Cremations have traditionally been performed by Hindus in Trinidad, as in India, on an open pyre of combustible wood. There has recently been established a gas fired, furnace type facility near the capital city of Port of Spain, but by far most of the cremations done are on the banks of the Caroni river in the north and at the estuary of the Godineau river in the south where this river enters the Gulf of Paria. The southern location is very picturesque, and the grounds are conspicuously well landscaped and impeccably maintained. The site is some thirty feet above water level and commands a panorama, extending clockwise across the Gulf of Venezuela, the Bocas, the Northern Range, the Central Plain, the oil refinery of Pointe-a-Pierre, San Fernando, the coastal highway, the mangrove swampland and in the immediate foreground the Godineau bridge.

Its signboards carry the appropriate legend both in English and Hindi, 'Shore of Peace' and 'Shanti Tiram'. The signboard was originally embellished with the Christian cross, the Muslim star and crescent, and the Hindu Aum, but it was quickly realised that Muslims do not cremate their dead, and the star and crescent were promptly erased.

There are certain stringent legal requirements associated with cremations: as with all deaths, a certificate of cause of death must be issued by a medical practitioner, this is taken to the Registrar of Births and Deaths who issues a death certificate based on the information on the doctor's certificate. At this stage, the deceased may be either interred or cremated. If the relatives decide to adopt the latter course, an application is made to the Police Superintendent of the District on a prescribed form, and he supplies two forms of certificate, one for the doctor who has issued the original cause of death certificate, and the other for an independent doctor who is not the regular medical attendant of the deceased. Both doctors then view the body independently (if one of them has not already done so), fill out the forms, and these are taken back to the police official who then issues a certificate of permission to cremate. The reasoning behind these procedures is to ensure that the person did not die as a result of foul play or of neglect. A final form is then given to the relative to be completed after cremation by a police officer confirming that the cremation has been performed according to plan.

At the cremation site meanwhile, a wooden pyre has been constructed some ten feet by three feet wide and six feet high. The body is placed inside the pile, an adequate space having been left during construction. Ghee and other inflammable substances are poured over the body. A close relative – preferably the eldest son if available – walks around the pyre five times then places a piece of camphor between the lips of the deceased, and, setting this alight, he initiates the cremation ceremony.

After about half an hour, the pyre is fully ablaze, and occasionally, with the contracture of the flexor muscles of the deceased, the body may be seen to raise its arms or even to sit up in a final gesture of adieu.

Total combustion takes several hours, and, with the winds of the Gulf of Paria sweeping over the site, the pyre may glow and burst spasmodically into flames throughout the night.

In the morning the relatives sweep up the ashes. Christians normally collect the fragments of charred bones and the ashes contiguous to them, for burial in their family plot in the cemetery, and Hindus, following the time-honoured custom brought by their ancestors from India, sweep the ashes of their departed into the waters to be dispersed far and wide along the shores of all the continents of the globe.

Smoking

When I was President of the Trinidad and Tobago Medical Association, there were two doctors on the executive committee whose smoking resembled that of the Usine Ste Madeline sugar factory which burned bagasse as a no-cost fuel.

For many years I had objected to smoking at meetings – to no avail. One doctor remarked that before we tried to put a stop to human smoking, we should attack the much greater polluter, the motor vehicles, since these machines produced several times more noxious gases than the poor maligned human smokers did. My reply, that we did not allow motor cars in our conference room, did not convince him and he remained of the same opinion.

At any rate, a motion was put before the committee that smoking should be prohibited in the conference room. It was passed by a majority of ten to two!

The following is an article by me which was published in the *Trinidad Guardian* of 6th June 1979.

SMOKING IN PUBLIC SHOULD BE BANNED

Tobacco is a poisonous plant which has displaced, from fertile land in Trinidad and other parts of the world, many useful food crops including members of its own family – the Solanaceae, for example the tomato, the melongene and the pepper.

Farmers are actually subsidised in order to propagate this toxic interloper. Advertising agencies grow rich from pushing this dope, and, irony of ironies, cigarette manufacturers are permitted to sponsor open air sports as if these salves of conscience, with accompanying salvos of publicity, can alleviate the years of suffering caused by cigarette-induced lung cancer, stroke and heart disease.

Tobacco smoke poisons all who breathe it, not only the smoker. At the most charitable it is a public nuisance. At worst, it is slow murder and suicide. There is no controversy about its position as an environmental pollutant – much more than littering, excessive noise or obscene language, yet its status in our society remains within the bounds of legality.

It is clearly immoral that smokers have the right to pollute public places at will with their noxious fumes, in the sense that these fumes can kill non-smokers, yet there is no law which prevents them from doing so. On private premises the owner can stop anyone from smoking if he wishes.

All these facts and observations have been known and made for a long time. Why, therefore, has such a necessary and fundamental law not been passed?

In order to answer this question, we must first of all consider that laws are passed in order to give the impression to the voters that Government is acting in the best interests of those who would vote for it, and sometimes laws are actually in the best interests of most or indeed all of the population. Government cannot therefore antagonise those who smoke and the long chain of people who retail, wholesale, sponsor and manufacture cigarettes and even matches, plus those who deal in the paper, printing, wood and other things at home and abroad, plus those who plant the tobacco here and abroad.

The vested interests are enormous and Government needs their votes in order to stay in power.

Before the OPEC-induced boom, the revenue from its taxation was an important factor in Government inaction regarding this homicidal product.

A third, important, but not widely recognised factor is the very real tranquillising effect of smoking: its hand movements, its nicotine and carbon monoxide content, and its satisfying Freudian sexual symbolism. These are useful things for voters faced with the endlessly unmitigated frustrations of an incompetent regime obsessed with appearances, placebos and placations.

It is likely that cigarettes, alcohol and non-taxed marijuana have reduced by more than 75% the number of placard-bearing demonstrators around Whitehall!

There is a gallant but small band of concerned citizens which has objected to cigarette advertising in certain places. This is not a giant step, but not ungallant either. Why not ban smoking itself, as well as advertising, in these places?

A law against smoking in public places would provide one arm of a pincer movement to rescue our young people from premature suffering and death. The second arm is the behaviour in private of those who detest the habit. Perhaps, if I write what I do, it might help:

I am sometimes polite when someone starts to smoke. I say: "Now, let me see which way the air is moving." I then get up from my chair and select another, or move my chair to the windward side of the smoker and say loudly, "Ah, now I cannot get the smoke!"

Of course some smokers are themselves polite and do what they always should, that is to say, they ask before lighting up: "May I smoke?" My reply is just as polite: "No."

But occasionally, as when my own grown up children have been smoking in the house before I arrive, I shout, "Who stink up the place? If all you want to kill youself (sic) with cancer and heart attacks is all you business, but do it outside and if you damn ass friends want to do it let them stink up their own house!"

In my office waiting room I have a multi-coloured sign garnished with the head of a wizened smoker, and at the top of his spiral of smoke a skull and crossbones. The inscription in three-inch letters reads: **'SMOKING IN GALLERY ONLY'**. The gallery is an open veranda abutting the pavement, and I hope that the law against smoking in public places is soon passed and that my veranda will be deemed a public place so as to effectively close the jaws of the pincer!

Yet we must realise that people smoke, not to annoy us or to kill us or themselves, but simply because they enjoy doing so. Thousands of volumes have been written on the psychological and other reasons for this, and the smoker must have our sympathy and tolerance as well as our condemnation – in the same manner and to the same degree that we exhibit these noble sentiments for the carriers of typhoid, tuberculosis or venereal disease.

*

This 1979 article – not surprisingly – had no impact, except a few phone calls expressing their admiration and deep sympathy for me! In May 1993, however, a resolution was moved in the Senate – the Upper House of our Parliament – by a member of the Opposition calling for a total ban of smoking in public places. Few Senators spoke on the resolution, most of them against the banning. This apathy provoked the following letter by me published in the *Guardian* of 9th May, 1993:

WHY ARE THE SENATORS SO SILENT?

I am disgusted by the timidity of most of the Senators on the motion calling for the banning of smoking in public places. I am particularly disappointed by the contribution of my former senatorial and present agricultural colleague, Professor Spence. Does he seriously believe that any agency – including any government – can afford the expense of an educational (i.e. an advertising) campaign which can effectively compete with the overwhelmingly rich tobacco companies?

The only solution for this nauseating, criminally prevalent and selfish habit is legislation for totally banning smoking in public places.

I would go further and call for the banning of advertisements for tobacco and alcohol in all our media.

Why were the Senators so silent? (At this point I had included the question, "Have they all got shares in the tobacco company?" This sentence was omitted in the published version!)

Let them realise that a local cigarette company has already seen the writing on the wall and has invested in a massive horticultural programme. This is a project which I am sure will receive the wholehearted approbation of my agricultural colleague. His job, and that of the other senators, should be to hasten the day when this disease-producing and nauseating habit will be replaced by the fragrance and beauty of tropical flowers.

Note: The motion, defeated, went up in smoke!

Race Relations

The inhabitants of Trinidad and Tobago are about 45% of African extraction, about 45% of East Indian origin and the remaining 10% are of Chinese, Semitic, Arawak and European ancestry. There has been a great deal of racial mixing, perhaps 25% of the population have ancestors of two or three races. One beautiful young lady of my acquaintance incorporates the genes of French, Spanish, Scottish, Carib, African and Indian forebears.

Our medical tradition, both in government practice and privately, has always been to give equally competent attention to all persons who come to us, regardless of race or religion. There are doctors of all races and religions in our country, and each one attends to representatives of every race. There is a vague preference on the part of the patient for a doctor of his own race, but generally, availability, competence, professional attitude and scale of fees are the characteristics which determine the patient's choice of doctor. In my own case, I was brought up in a home in which my schoolmaster father, by his own example, taught us to regard all races as equal and entitled to equality of respect. One striking example of this in practice, was his attention to the feet of pupils whom he regularly lined up, selected all those with chigoes and sores, and skilfully treated all of them, regardless of race, religion class or caste. Side by side stood Brahmins, Chamars, Muslims and Africans, all fellow pupils and fellow patients of this kind and fatherly gentleman.

It therefore, came naturally to me, in attending to patients, to be almost oblivious as to their race and colour, but in Trinidad no one can ever be completely unaware of these obvious characteristics and not react – even unconsciously – to the colonial heritage of accepting the superiority of white over brown and black. In effect, everyone is race and colour conscious and as it happens sometimes even prejudiced, but most persons will not descend to discrimination in public on that basis. To my everlasting shame, I was once caught out in a manner which I would never before have thought possible.

A lovely English girl came into my examination room with her two beautiful boys aged six and four. They had a mild bronchitis which they had contracted during their month in glorious Tobago, mainly on the enchanting coral beach and crystal waters of Pigeon Point. They were all superbly tanned, the boys more so than their mother. When I had finished she asked what the fee was. I told her ten dollars (this was before the oil boom).

"Okay," she said, "My husband will come in and pay."

As they went through the door leading to the waiting room, a very dark man – apparently of African extraction and in a hurry – tried to squeeze past them and enter the examination room.

"Oh, excuse me," I said to him. "Just a minute please, the lady's husband has to come in."

"I am her husband," he replied.

I could have dropped through the floor. Unsuspected by my rational self, I had been betrayed by my colour consciousness which lay treacherously just below the surface in my mind. How could I ever have assumed that the beautifully tanned children were the beneficiaries merely of the ultra violet, and not attribute at least some of their burnished glow to the genes of a noble ancestry?

The Private Practitioners
Advisory Committee

On the initiative of Dr Max Awon, a prominent and popular obstetrician-gynaecologist, who was elected to parliament and appointed Minister of Health, a committee was convened with the following terms of reference:

1. To provide a forum for discussions between the Minister and Private Practitioners.
2. To enable the Minister to keep the private sector of the profession informed of important developments in the health policy of the nation and the proposals for their implementation.
3. To provide the private sector of the profession with an opportunity to express their views on health matters generally and to advise on measures for improvement of the health services.
4. To discuss the possibilities for participation of private practitioners in the health services of the Ministry.
5. Any other relevant matters.

The first meeting was held on 8th November 1967, and on 28th November Dr Awon wrote inviting me to serve on the committee. At the meeting of 5th December, the following persons attended.

Dr Max Awon (Chairman), Dr L.M. Commissiong, Dr Robert Gunness, Dr J. Millar, Dr Horace Beckford, Dr Ivan Perot, Dr Ewing Chow, Dr Hilda Bynoe, Dr B. Chang Pong, Dr Aldwyn G. Francis, Dr Sir Henry Pierre, Dr Martin Sampath, Dr I. Sears-Carter, Mr J. Bynoe (by special invitation as an architect to advise on the re-modelling of the Casualty department) and Mr Trevor Romano (Secretary).

Meetings were held monthly and were extremely interesting and informative. They certainly did justice to the terms of reference, as evidenced by the following sample list of subjects we discussed.

Improvement of hospital casualty departments
Dental 'quacks'
Structure of the health services
Shortage of doctors: (Discussion of a lead paper by myself!)
Immunisation programmes
The Clinmobile
Doctors' and nurses' accommodation and residence
Domiciliary midwifery
Paramedical personnel
A National Health Plan
Decentralisation of health services
Upgrading of immunisation record cards
The value and risk of Pertussis immunisation
Health hazard posed by stray dogs
Dental auxiliaries
Entitlement to private consulting practice by Government doctors
Work permits for non-national doctors
Complaints from the public about treatment at Government
    Institutions
Mistakes in a Parliamentary Bill regarding dispensing doctors
Scholarships as incentive for recruiting doctors
Information to relatives about in-patients in hospitals
Congratulations to Dr Hilda Bynoe (one of our Committee
    members) on her appointment as Governor of Grenada.

The fifteenth and last meeting was held on 25th February, 1970. In this month and in March, the country was in turmoil, following an army mutiny and militant 'Black Power' activities. On April 21st, a State of Emergency was declared with dawn to dusk curfew. All operations of the committee were suspended and have never been resumed.

Several changes and improvements in medical services were made as a result of our discussions, and Dr Awon is to be congratulated on his initiative. It is to be hoped that future Ministers of Health will follow his example.

AIDS and Sexual Transmission

The latest available figures reveal that one thousand, five hundred people in Trinidad and Tobago are suffering from AIDS; this is 0.1% of our population. There is widespread publicity seeking to educate the public about the dangers and about ways of preventing infection, for example, abstinence, single partner and the use of condoms. Many more HIV positives occur among persons of African descent than among persons of East Indian descent. Various hypotheses have been advanced to account for this, for example, the use of curry, and genetic resistance.

In the following article, published in the *Caribbean Medical Journal*, Volume 15, Nos 1&2 of 1953, I discussed my findings relating to the incidence of Syphilis-positive patients, and it appears that a similar situation could be existing with reference to AIDS:

The Influence of Socio-Anthropological Factors on the Incidence of Syphilis in a Heterogenous Group of Pregnant Women in Trinidad

Trinidad has a population of six hundred thousand, of whom half are negroes and one-third are East Indian.

San Fernando is the chief town of South Trinidad, and to the Colonial Hospital there come patients from the entire south of the Island.

At the ante-natal clinic of this institution the opportunity presented itself of analysing a series of consecutive cases of normal women who, having had intercourse, had exposed themselves to possible contact with syphilis: this study also gives some indication of the incidence of syphilis among the male population of this area. This particular group, viz. pregnant women with its obvious family associations, is of particular moment, and this will become more apparent as the discussion proceeds.

INCIDENCE OF SYPHILIS

A total of 2,246 consecutive cases were qualitatively Kahn tested between June 1951 and October 1952. Of these, a hundred and thirty-one gave a positive reaction, that is 5.8%. When these cases were classified, according to race and with reference to geographical distribution, the following results were obtained:

GROUP		TOTAL NO.	KAHN POSITIVE	% KAHN POSITIVE
East Indians				
	Town	218	7	3.2%
	Country	1070	28	2.6%
Negroes				
	Town	467	58	12.4%
	Country	491	38	7.7%

All persons living within the official boundaries of the Borough of San Fernando are classified as town cases.

Women attended the clinic in roughly the same proportions as they exist in the area. In the town there are more Negroes than East Indians, while in the environs, East Indians are overwhelmingly more numerous. Although there is a substantial degree of social intercourse between the two races, there is only a little sexual intercourse between them, whether casual, in concubinage or in marriage.

COMPARISON OF TOWN AND COUNTRY

There is markedly more syphilis in the town than in the country among both races. This is in accord with the results of similar studies in all parts of the world, and the reason usually given is that there is more promiscuity in the town. While San Fernando is not at present a flourishing seaport, it has the status of being an important centre of communications and business in the south of the island.

COMPARISON OF NEGROES AND EAST INDIANS

There is considerably more syphilis among Negroes than among East Indians both in town and country. The probable causes for this makes an interesting study in social anthropology. There are striking contrasts in the development and evolution of family life, and in cultural attitudes between these two groups since they first arrived from their respective homelands.

It will never be known for certain whether the Negroes and East Indians brought syphilis with them from Africa and India respectively. It is most unlikely that they received it from the aborigines of Trinidad, because on their arrival, the aborigines were already almost extinct. While it is uncertain that fifteenth century Americans were the source of European syphilis, there is little doubt that Negroes and East Indians in Trinidad obtained most of theirs from the European planters in the Island.

CONTRASTS IN EVOLUTION OF FAMILY LIFE

The Negro family as a unit suffered considerable disruption during the period of slavery. At emancipation, cohabitation rather than marriage was the rule, and a fairly loose association between man and woman has been their legacy. This has been modified through the influence of the Christian church, so that there exist, at present, four types of families:

(a) The formal family based on marriage and approximating the Christian family in other parts of the world (Simey calls this the 'Christian Family').

(b) Faithful concubinage with no legal status, but well established and enduring for at least three years.

(c) The compassionate family in which the partners live together for pleasure and convenience and usually for less than three years.

(d) The disintegrate family, consisting of a woman and her children, usually severally fathered with occasional visits from former and prospective fathers.

These four stations are in themselves not permanent, and a single woman may in her lifetime change her status throughout these classifications and back again. The original association is probably most commonly that of the compassionate family, and this may evolve through the period of faithful concubinage with the same or a different partner into a Christian marriage with the children and occasionally the grandchildren attending the formal ceremony. Social dynamics have therefore been, for a very long time, almost ideal for the rapid dissemination of syphilis among Negroes.

In contrast, East Indians, when originally brought to work on the plantations, arrived, in general, in family units, and there has never been any widespread disruption in the close association between man and woman living in a family. There was also very little, if any, disruption in the religious and social customs of these immigrants. Among both Hindus and Muslims, the accent has always been on early and lifelong marriage to one partner: among those Muslims who were polygamous, to one male partner. Since the family associations listed above as (b), (c) and (d) are to be found among East Indians only to a relatively small extent, the opportunity for the spread of syphilis has been limited.

EFFECT OF FAMILY DISORGANISATION ON THE CHILD, AND ON SEXUAL BEHAVIOUR

Among Negroes, the looseness of family structure and relative lack of restraint and discipline has had a direct influence on the attitude of the child towards its physiological functions, including sex. The child is not fed regularly, except when it cries, and usually it must cry loudly and persistently before being fed. It develops the habit of performing its functions as soon as possible after the biological demand is evident and of making its demands in a tone of urgency. This attitude finds its way naturally into sex, and the Negro is sexually an aggressive person. The general lack of close association with a father results in the absence of Oedipus/Electra complexes among Negroes in Trinidad.

Among East Indians, the rigid, patriarchal, family unit at once imposes a strong discipline on the child. His desires are more easily fulfilled by submissiveness than by aggressiveness, and in general not only are his economic problems identified with and controlled by his father's family and greater family, but his conjugal associations as well. The Oedipus and Electra complexes are so well developed among East Indians, as often to be of psycho-pathological importance in his adaptation to the Western way of life.

It is unfortunate that research has not yet been done in Trinidad along the lines followed by Kinsey in the United States. The general impression is that Negroes in Trinidad are more promiscuous than East Indians, and this would be the natural result of the forces at work outlined above.

(The Socio-anthropological discussion is based on Hugh Sampath's *Negro Personality and West Indian Culture* Columbia University Project 1950 and T.S. Simey 1945, *Welfare and Planning in the West Indies*.)

Homosexuals

Although I know very many male and a few female homosexuals socially, though not participatorily, only a few male adherents have been my patients.

One of these, a handsome young man of twenty-five, had a severe bladder infection which responded very well to a standard sulphamethoxazole-trimethoprim combination tablet. All doctors know that the causative B. coli organism, besides being abundant in the rectum, also occurs almost naturally in the nearby female organ, and I was not at first concerned about the source of his infection. But he returned within two months with the same condition. This time I treated him with Noroxin and he again made a dramatic recovery. When he returned shortly after, again re-infected, I knew that I was missing something and asked him whether he was homosexual. He replied that he was, and had been sexually active in this manner for many years. I explained how his re-infections were brought about, and recommended the use of a condom. He in turn told me that this would be difficult, even with the customary lubricant, since the anus, unlike the female introitus, gave little room for manoeuvre. Very sadly, a blood test showed this young man to be HIV positive. He contracted pneumonia two years later and died.

I remember some of the remarks included in a vote of thanks I once delivered to Dr Courtney Bartholomew, Professor of Medicine at our local Medical School, on the occasion of his AIDS lecture to the Medical Association.

"There is a great deal of condemnation in some quarters of homosexual practices, and the dogma abounds that AIDS is divine punishment for homosexuals. But it seems to me that since the virus appears to enter the minute cracks in the anus, which is much more susceptible to cracking than the vulva, AIDS in homosexuals is a question of skin rather than sin!"

I read recently that there is a genetic factor involved in the development of homosexuality. While this may be so, my own discussions with both homosexuals and heterosexuals lead me to theorise that early sexual contacts between little boys and girls must be a potent determining factor. Most heterosexuals had their first sexual experience – of however limited and non-penetrating a nature – with a member of the opposite sex, and nearly, if not all, homosexuals got their first sexual experience very late in life and with a member of the same sex.

A few doctors tell me that they remember having sexual 'intercourse' of an incomplete character at ages ranging from six to nine, at which time the act was fairly well performed, even resulting in an orgasm! They add that after these experiences they could never imagine how any male person could prefer the dry, hard anus to what they describe as the delectably soft, moist, tender feminine part.

I recently saw this topic discussed in a television series called *The Nature of Things* with David Suzuki, and their findings appear to confirm the deductions above.

After all this, one must admit that physical sexual function is not the only incentive for homosexual liaisons, in the same way that sexual intercourse is not the only event which attracts and keeps together heterosexual partners, in some instances literally 'till death do us part'.

Family Relationships

Most Trinbagonians speak English, and the names by which they refer to their relatives follow the established English pattern. Persons of East Indian descent often define their relatives much more accurately, necessitated in the first instance by the presence under one roof of numerous levels of corresponding relationships in the greater family, and the need to be specific in referring to any one of them.

The following is a list of such relationships, a list which I do not, by any means, presume to be complete:

RELATIONSHIP	ENGLISH	HINDI
Father	Father, papa, dad, pater	Baph, pitaji
Mother	Mother, mama, mater	Mai, mataji
Son	Son	Bayta
Daughter	Daughter	Baytee
Brother	Brother	Bhaiya
His wife	Sister-in-law	Bhowjie
Sister (elder)	Sister	Deedya
Sister (any)	Sister	Bahin
Sister's husband	Brother-in-law	Banoi
Father's elder brother	Uncle	Dada
His wife	Aunt	Dadee
Father's younger brother	Uncle	Kāka, Chācha
His wife	Aunt	Kākee, Chāchee
Mother's brother	Uncle	Mamoo
His wife	Aunt	Mamee
Mother's sister	Aunt	Mousie
Her husband	Uncle	Mousa
Father's sister	Aunt	Phuwa

Her husband	Uncle	Poopha
Father's father	Grandfather	Ajah
Father's mother	Grandmother	Ajee
Mother's father	Grandfather	Nana
Mother's mother	Grandmother	Nanee
Two brothers' wives	Sisters-in-law	Barkee (the elder) Chotkee (the younger)
Two sisters' husbands	Brothers-in-law	Sarobhai
Son's wife	Daughter-in-law	Bahoo
Daughter's husband	Son-in-law	Damad, junwaie
Couple's fathers		Samdhi
Couple's mothers		Samdhin
Two wives of one man		(Combos)[6] Santin
Husband	Husband	Patee
Wife	Wife	Patnee
Grandson	Grandson	Natee
Granddaughter	Granddaughter	Natin

---

6 Local English

My Prostitute Patients

These ladies reveal their professions to me quite openly, without embarrassment and even with pride. Some of them seek treatment for a sexually transmitted disease, this being their occupational hazard, but most of their illnesses are what any doctor, lawyer, priest or labourer would normally have.

One of these, a pretty girl of thirty, had been in the business since the age of fifteen. For her first intimate performance she was paid one shilling. Those were sterling days: although dollars were the common currency, we had half-penny copper coins worth one cent, a penny coin of the same metal worth two cents, a tiny three-penny silver piece valued at six cents, a silver six-penny coin worth twelve cents, and the following all in silver: one shilling – twenty-four cents, two shillings – forty-eight cents (also called a 'florin'), half-a-crown or 'two and six' worth sixty cents. Our paper money was in dollars: a red one dollar note, and a blue two dollars were issued by the Government of Trinidad and Tobago while fives and tens were issued by several commercial banks in various shades of green with individual designs and known as 'bank notes'.

At that time, only two professional groups used the sterling system in their day by day (or night by night) transactions; the other was the legal profession – thought to be the third oldest. The second oldest – the doctors, being always the most practical and thoughtful, had in Trinidad and Tobago already switched to dollars.

King's Counsels (under George V) charged their clients in guineas, that is, twenty-one shillings or five dollars and four cents. The magistrate fined his unsuccessful defendants in pounds and shillings, and the litigant quickly made a mental calculation and paid in dollars and cents: one pound at that time being four dollars and eighty cents. The expression that our dollar was 'tied to Sterling' was a reality in more ways than one.

Now to get back to the subject of our heading – and to point out its relevance to the above discourse on financial equivalents.

Our local calypsonians, who dealt with every subject under the sun, moon and stars – serious and salacious – have traced the general inflationary trend in our economy, as reflected in prostitutes' emoluments.

At the time of our young heroine's initiation, one such bard sang:

"If you can't stand the digging
Gimme back me shilling."

A later calypsonian's song commemorated both the inflation and the accepted change in currency thus:

"Myra, Myra, the boat in the harbour
Drop you bloomers and f--- for you dollar."

During World War II, when the Americans were building their Army Base at Waller field at the North Centre of Trinidad and their Navy Base at Point Cumana, west of Port of Spain, one of our very famous singers, the 'Lord Invader' crooned thus:

"Every mother and daughter
Down at Point Cumana
Working for the Yankee dollar."

The US dollar was worth $1.10 Trinidad and Tobago currency at that time.

When our subject first came to see me, her going fee for each occasion was ten dollars. She intimated that she charged young boys half price, since it required little activity on her part – the act in most instances almost completing itself, resulting in a much quicker turnover.

This young lady came to me for several non-sexual ailments for many years, and only once for a venereal disease which responded quickly to antibiotic therapy. She came much later with a long standing cough; the chest signs pointed to tuberculosis at a time when this disease had become a rarity in the country. X-ray and sputum were positive and I sent her to the Caura Chest Hospital in North

Trinidad. She made a complete recovery and when she brought her child to me one year later, she told me she had retired from her profession, and now she and her husband were running a successful snackette.

The Country Haven

This was the name of a thriving brothel near Siparia, and the star hostesses were from Colombia on the South American mainland. Several of these ladies came to me for a wide variety of ailments, again, seldom for a sexually transmitted condition. One of them, a very charming person who spoke English fluently, gave me a great deal of information about the activities at the Haven. It seems that they catered for all classes and races of clients: their practice of democracy was enviable, and there were also African and East Indian ladies in their entourage. The standard fee for Colombian companionship was fifty dollars, for East Indian: forty dollars and for an African: thirty dollars. When she told me this, I was reminded of a joke told to us at dinner by a Kenyan surgeon in Nairobi, in 1983.

A certain visitor to Kenya, anxious to sample that country's offerings, asked a prostitute her price. "Ten pounds," she quoted.

"But all over Europe they ask for only five pounds!" he expostulated.

"Well," she retorted, "that was Common Market. This here is 'Black Market!'"

The Country Haven prospered for many years during the oil boom, but tragically it burned to the ground a few years ago. One patient, a neighbour of the establishment, described the holocaust.

"It was horrible. The building was blazing, the ground floor was completely engulfed, and the women were upstairs in their rooms screaming piteously for help at the windows. There was no escape as the stairs were in flames. Some of them jumped blazing to the ground writhing in agony before they lost consciousness and died. No one was saved."

When I heard this story I was overwhelmed with sadness and with pity. I kept remembering the young lady who had told me so much about the haven. Was she one of those who fell in flaming agony that night? May their souls rest in peace.

Red Light and Locations

In the smaller villages and towns there are no recognised 'Red Light Districts'. In the capital city of Port of Spain, the location for these pleasurable activities is George Street. This port of the Spaniards had several parallel streets, each one starting at the waterfront – later 'Marine' and now 'Independence' Square, and running northwards towards what is now Queen's Park Savannah. One of these is Abercromby[7] Street, named after the English admiral who captured the island from the Spaniards. East of this is Chacon Street, retaining the name of the Spanish Governor who capitulated to Abercromby, and eastward in order are streets named after English royalty: Frederick, Henry, Charlotte and George.

George developed into the city's red light district, on account of easy access from the waterfront to both the street and its residents.

In San Fernando, our smaller city, the street leading from the waterfront towards the hill and the hinterland was High Street which ended at the junction of Pointe-a-Pierre Road and Coffee Street. Leading away from this junction is Mucurapo Street. 'Mucurapo' is an Amerindian word meaning 'silk cotton tree'. This street, in the days of small sugar plantations, separated the Belle Vue plantation on the East from the Paradise plantation on the west, so that silk-cotton, in effect, united a lovely view with paradise!

---

[7] This original spelling still survives in a signboard on a wall bordering the street.

Scorpion Stings
and Snake Bites

Scorpion stings are fairly common at the start of the rainy season – usually from May to June. It seems that these arachnids hide in widespread cracks in the shrinking clay soil of the preceding dry season, and come into buildings when these cracks become flooded. Many schools have to be closed to students for up to two weeks at this time in order to get rid of these animals by spraying. Reactions to these stings are very unpredictable: some may result simply in pain at the site of penetration for a few hours, others may have intractable vomiting with severe epigastric pain, others may suffer cardiac arrest and die. Small children are the ones who are most likely to have severe or fatal reactions. My standard treatment is an intra-muscular injection of cortisone or a related steroid, sweet drinks, complete bed rest under the covers, and close observation for six hours, which is the critical period.

I have seen delayed occurrences of pancrealitis and cyst formation, but never after steroids have been given early.

We have three very poisonous snakes in Trinidad and many non-poisonous one. There are no snakes of any kind in Tobago. We have two Bushmaster species, the Mappipire zanana and M. balsin, and we have the universally known coral snake. At one time we imported snake and scorpion anti-serum from the Butanan company at Sao Paulo in Brazil, but these were not specific to our snakes and scorpions, and reactions to their horse globulins became too common for the continued use of these sera.

Fortunately, unlike scorpion stings, snake bites are today quite uncommon.

We have a very large Boa constrictor which bites like a dog and can cause mechanical damage, but this species is non-venomous. Our

Huila, which lives in our swamp waters, has been known to crush and swallow calves and goats.

As an interesting aside: the Cocrico, one of our national and protected birds – the size of a large chicken – is abundant in Tobago but does not exist in Trinidad. The Cocrico lays its eggs on the ground or on bushes near to the ground. It is thought that these eggs can mature safely in Tobago because there are no snakes there to prey on them!

The 'Jharray' Ritual

This age old practice is usually performed by persons of East Indian origin, very often as a first line of treatment for a wide variety of ailments, including jaundice, scorpion stings, snake bites, marasmus, convulsions, vomiting and shingles.

There are certain beliefs, associated with some illnesses, which have a bearing on the performance of this ritual. It is commonly believed, for example, that 'Bad Eye', called 'Najar' in Hindi and in French Patois 'Maljo' (a derivation of 'Mal des yeux'), is responsible for listlessness, loss of appetite, abdominal pain and vomiting in children. Many of these recover immediately after jharraying.

'Malkadi' means convulsions – a corruption of 'Mal que dieu' or 'God given' – in much the same way as doctors describe certain illnesses, the aetiology of which we are ignorant, as 'idiopathic'. Again, the convulsions may cease after jharraying. 'Pallai' – the rapid movement of the abdominal muscles as a result of strong diaphragmatic breathing when asthma or pneumonia has struck a child, is frequently jharrayed. Asthmatic 'pallai' often stops dramatically during jharraying, especially when the location of the ritual is some distance from that in which the attack first occurred. Jaundice is often visibly reduced with the repetition of the ritual week by week. Some scorpion stings and snake bites (especially by non-poisonous snakes) have no untoward effects at all after jharraying, but some stings and some venomous snake bite victims deteriorate after the procedure, and it is felt that these patients waited too long before applying to the jharrayer.

Although it is well known in medical circles that many of the above conditions disappear spontaneously, it would be unwise for any of us to pooh-pooh the practice, since the procedure is usually accompanied by prayer, itself excellent adjuvant therapy.

Jharraying takes many forms. The two commonest ones are:

Use of Cocoyea Sticks

These sticks are the slender, firm ribs of the leaves of the coconut palm, and an extremely effective broom made of about a hundred of these sticks can be found at any time in most rural homes in Trinidad. Two sticks[8] of exactly equal lengths – about twenty-four to thirty-six inches – are held together at one pair of ends, the other ends are manipulated to touch the patient gently from forehead to toes seven times, slowly, and each time the far ends are allowed to touch the ground. After this is done, the sticks are measured. If the condition suspected is present, one of the sticks is observed to be shorter. This is diagnostic jharraying for suspected cases of the 'Evil Eye', and the procedure is also believed to be curative.

Use of Devil's Grass

In cases of jaundice, the instrument used is Devil's Grass which is dipped in mustard oil before each pass over the body. It has been reported that as the jaundice gradually leaves the body, the mustard oil becomes thicker in consistency.

Use of Viboutie

This is the ash from burnt offerings, consisting of black till, rice, googool, incense, camphor and ghee. A bit of the ashes is held between the thumb and the index and middle fingers, and placed on the forehead of the patient. This is accompanied by solemn prayers.

As mentioned above, jharraying is regarded as the first line of attack on the illness, the relatives almost invariably pursue the second line, namely a visit to an orthodox medical practitioner, or more accurately, an exponent of standard medical practices.

---

[8] Bringing with them, symbolically, the cleansing function of the cocoyea broom.

Mango Leaves and the Mango

These leaves are also commonly used in jharraying, and the wood is popular as the fuel for burnt offerings. This is not unexpected as the plant is from India, the botanical name being *Mangifera Indica*. Its delicious fruit, appropriately called 'The king of tropical fruits', has innumerable varieties. The latex of most of these fruits can come into contact with the skin to no effect, but I have seen slight blistering of the forearm in a young girl, caused by the exudate from a not fully ripe 'starch' variety of mango. This plant belongs to the same botanical family, *Anacardiacae*, as the cashew, which is *Anacardium occidentale*, an American plant. Here, the cashew nut is the fruit, and I have seen very severe blistering of the mouth, lips and face in children who have bitten this fruit in its raw state. The skin of most unripe mangoes can be bitten, chewed or eaten raw with complete safety.

The Trinidad and Tobago Medical Association

(Presented at the Commonwealth Medical Conference held in Nicosia, Cyprus, on 5th October, 1986, by Dr Carl Lee. Written by me, as Past President, Trinidad and Tobago Medical Association)

The Trinidad and Tobago Medical Association has the distinction of having enjoyed complete democracy and almost complete autonomy for several decades before Trinidad and Tobago herself.

It started in 1892 as a branch of the British Medical Association, adopting all the democratic and self-determining traditions of that body, and it maintained these characteristics after the severance of this umbilical attachment on the attainment of independence by the nation in 1962. The Association has retained the strongest affiliation with the parent body.

In marked contrast, Trinidad and Tobago, originally inhabited by Arawaks and Caribs (recalled today largely by the many euphonious place names they left behind), had been separate colonies of several European nations since the end of the fifteenth century. It would be no exaggeration to say that for nearly five centuries these islands experienced naked imperialism and racism with their corollaries of discrimination by race, colour, class, caste and religion. The need for cheap labour on the sugar plantations stimulated the importation of slaves from Africa and indentured labourers from India, so that today the descendants of these two groups each constitute 40% of the islands' population, with peoples originating in every continent of the globe making up the remaining 20%, largely through genetic recombination

This heterogeneous mass, of about one and a quarter million souls on two thousand square miles of land, being the two southernmost islands of the Caribbean chain, sitting a mere seven miles off the north-eastern shore of South America, is today an independent democracy with a Westminster system of Government, a British legal system, 90% literacy in English – the official language – adult franchise and every person, male and female, equal before the law.

But old habits and prejudices die hard, so that unpleasant rivalry based illogically on race, colour, religion and social class, occasionally raises its ugly head and is always a factor to be considered as lying just beneath the surface. In this milieu, our Association, because of its long standing democratic and independent tradition, and also because social mobility in Trinidad and Tobago is a remarkable phenomenon by any standard in the world, flourishes like an oasis: our presidents have been European, African, Indian, Chinese, Arab and a variety of mixtures of these at various times, and their grandparents have been slaves, labourers, millionaire landowners and combinations of these. Our membership has always been a kaleidoscopic representation of the inhabitants of the country.

The Association takes a keen interest in the politics of the nation, but one of its inflexible traditions is that as an Association it never aligns itself with, nor supports any particular political party. As it happens, several of its presidents and officers have been active members of different parties: some have been ministers of government, others merely parliamentarians. On at least one occasion, an opposition politician has been a political prisoner, yet they have sat and counselled together on medical, political and medico-political matters, arriving hopefully at consensus or deciding by democratic vote on a concerted course of action.

In this connection, the following examples may be of interest:

The Public Order Bill

The Government published a Bill which sought to give to the police certain powers which the Association felt were unjustified. After discussion, it was decided by an overwhelming majority (a Government Minister was in the minority) that the Association should publish its stand against this legislation in the daily press. It so happened that there was a public outcry against the Bill and it was withdrawn.

130

Capital Punishment

The call to abolish capital punishment was hotly discussed at an Association meeting. The abolitionists lost the contest, only because there was a tie in the voting and the chairman declined to exercise his prerogative of a casting vote which would have changed the status quo.

Abortion 'On Demand'

The question of the legalisation of all forms of abortion raised a veritable hornet's nest. There was such a marked and emotionally charged difference of opinion that anything resembling consensus, compromise or even substantial majority was impossible. The Association therefore published a statement revealing the wide divergence of strongly held views among its members and explaining why, as an Association, a definite stand could not be taken. A decision based on a slim majority would have been quite meaningless.

The Air Pilots' Strike

During this strike it appeared to some that one or more of our members had been guilty of a breach of confidentiality by permitting the medical records of one of the pilots to be published. Indeed, intimate medical details were read out in Parliament by the then Minister of Industry and Commerce and broadcast by radio and television to the entire nation! The Association investigated and discussed the situation with two of the doctors concerned in attendance. It published its condemnation of the broadcast, but was satisfied that the two doctors themselves were not guilty of any breach of confidentiality.

The *Trinidad Guardian* published the following report:

The Trinidad and Tobago Medical Association has expressed concern about the public statements made in Parliament about the medical records of British West Indian Airways pilot Captain Malcolm Hernandez.

The Association wrote to the Speaker of the House of Representatives yesterday, re-emphasising the 'sacrosanct relationship between doctor and patient'. The Association drew attention to the 'wide implications' and asked, did the patient give permission for his medical records to be made public? Has Parliament now set for itself the precedent whereby any State-controlled enterprise may now make available to the House any confidential medical record by the enterprises medical officer, with or without his consent and that of the patient concerned?

The letter continued:

The Trinidad and Tobago Medical Association has reacted with displeasure, alarm and shock to the placing before Parliament, and the attendant broadcast to the nation, of the medical records of a patient on Friday, February 3, 1978.

We find it difficult to believe that any member of the medical profession would deliberately consent to, or condone, this practice. We have been assured by Professor C. Bartholomew and Professor M. Beaubrun that they were not in fact consulted about the release in Parliament.

While we are aware that Parliament is the highest authority in the land, and that a Court of Law can require medical records to be divulged before it in the interest of justice, even magistrates and judges often exercise – and are expected to exercise – their most highly considered discretion before adopting such a course; and then on occasion, certain disclosures are required to be made in chambers.

We recognise the existence of the Speaker's discretionary powers to prevent such disclosures in Parliament, despite the privileged position of proceedings in the House.

We are of the opinion that the medical records should not have been read in the House, and that the subsequent publication in the media was most unfortunate and indefensible.

Search of Doctors' Homes by the Police

Two of our doctors' homes were searched in quick succession ostensibly for arms and ammunition. The searches were fruitless, and drew an immediate rebuke from the Association. One victim sued, and received a substantial sum from the Government. Harassment ceased.

The Association is often called upon to advise, regarding some of Government's policies and projects, and to nominate members to Boards and Committees. We have always complied and cooperated, and we feel that these services are sincerely appreciated. There have been occasions, however, when our advice has been callously spurned: at the blueprint stage, we sought representation on the task force of a proposed multimillion dollar 'Mount Hope Medical Complex'. Our request was rejected. We then asked to meet and discuss with the task force. This was granted, and at this meeting we objected to various things, including the location of the complex. We were told that our objections were useless – that the entire matter was already decided. As it has transpired, there has been a multi-million dollar cost overrun, and the project now has the economic status of a ravenous white elephant.

While there is unlikely to be any overt threat to the independence of the Association, there is the real possibility of subtle forms of coercion: the awarding of National Honours to doctors who have not been openly critical of the regime, the withholding of such honours from doctors nominated by the Association at the express invitation of the Government, the covert promises (to members whose criticisms of Government have been too objective) of certain posts, have all been successfully employed.

The real strength of the Association lies in its economic independence. It is supported financially entirely by its members, it owns its own headquarters property, and has the goodwill of private pharmaceutical firms, who generously support many of its projects such as lectures, seminars and so on.

A very large proportion of its membership is comprised of private practitioners who do not depend on Government for their sustenance. Only its members can dictate its policy, and determine its course of action.

In sharp contrast, our young nation is, in theory, politically, but in practice, not economically, independent. So that, in Trinidad and Tobago, the two most potent guarantors of freedom for individuals and institutions are the legal system and the press.

The Legal System

Despite the changes following independence and the birth of our republic, the important judicial baby has not been 'thrown out with the bath water'. The legal system, including the right of appeal to the Privy Council, has been retained. There have been victories as well as defeats for the Government and its agencies at all levels, and these judgements have been accepted, albeit with a greater or lesser degree of grace by some parties.

Press Freedom

Both daily newspapers are open to public and editorial comment on all issues – from sport to politics, and from sport in politics to politics in sport! Editorial censorship is minimal and is usually explained by limitation of space. There is no official government censorship of any section of the media.

The electronic media (one television and two radio stations) give excellent coverage. The television and one radio station are Government owned, and are allegedly controlled by independent boards – but this allegation is often contested.

There are at least half a dozen weekly newspapers, some with widespread circulation and an avid readership. Most of these cater blatantly to public fascination for sensation, scandal, sex and sin. Neither boardroom nor bedroom is exempt from their attention. One of them, under new management and a more enlightened editorial policy, appears to be evolving into an accurate mirror of national events, and its stories often scoop by a fortnight those in the daily press. The Medical Association obtains its due share of attention. Doctors' behaviour in the examination room as well as bar room, is often probed by the finely honed lances of these ubiquitous cavaliers of the press.

Our Association publishes the *Caribbean Medical Journal* several times each year, as articles and advertising come in. Apart from strictly medical and scientific topics, the *CMJ* usually carries articles dealing with political, legal, economic and other matters impinging on the practice of medicine.

The retention of the right of appeal to the Privy Council has been interpreted as a symptom of political immaturity. In this regard, our nation has not presumed to wear an undeserved dignity. We hope, with the passage of time and the development of true maturity, that Caribbean peoples will speed the evolution of a Caribbean Court that possesses a prestige which will properly satisfy the need for a supreme judicial authority in the region.

It is with this kind of perspective that the Trinidad and Tobago Medical Association maintains and seeks to strengthen its links with other Caribbean medical associations. It does appear that similar institutions and Government Ministries involved in Law, Agriculture, Education, Engineering and so on, could, with considerable advantage to the future development of the Caribbean, do the same. Our links with Commonwealth medical associations – such as we again strengthen at this conference – constitute a wider step, and again this could profitably be emulated by institutions and Ministries of Government in other disciplines of endeavour. In this way, may we expand, step by tentative step, wave succeeding wave, like ever widening ripples in our global pond.

We professional men and women are a fortunate and highly privileged few, sprinkled like salt among a teeming mass of disadvantaged, hungry, suffering humanity. May we never lose our savour, for how then will humanity be salted?

Let us strive unceasingly, therefore, to quicken the pace of the movement forward – our goal must be clear: we must aim at nothing less than the universal enjoyment of health, wealth and happiness which is the just dessert of all who dwell on our bountiful planet Earth.

Ethical, Sociological and Political Aspects of the 1971-72 Poliomyelitis Epidemic in Trinidad

(Reprinted from Caribbean Medical Journal, *December 1973)*

This report, sent in by Dr M.S. Sampath, a member of a TTMA three-man Poliomyelitis Epidemic Sub-committee, is a minority one, as the other members of the committee[9] did not sign the report:

Historical Introduction

As a result of this epidemic, one hundred and eighty-four cases of paralysis were reported and thirteen persons died.

For some years there has been a Virus Research Laboratory in Trinidad, located at the University of the West Indies at Federation Park, one of whose functions has been to monitor the presence of viruses pathogenic to man. It has been the custom of the head of this unit to inform the relevant authority when, in his opinion, such incidence is significant in relation to public health.

Poliomyelitis vaccine, both of the monovalent and trivalent types, are readily available on short notice from manufacturers in North America and the United Kingdom. Three doses, at approximately monthly intervals, are usually regarded as adequate to give sufficient resistance to the disease.

---

[9] In the repressive political atmosphere at that time they were undoubtedly afraid of reprisal by the regime.

In March 1971, Dr Ardoin of the Virus Research Centre detected a significant increase in the wild poliomyelitis virus population, and reported his findings by telephone to the Ministry of Health. In June and July 1971, there were clinical cases reported in Venezuela, and Dr Santiago, Medical Officer of Health during the same months, having been informed of the presence of the wild virus in significant proportions in Trinidad, also reported it to the Ministry of Health.

In May 1971, the Trinidad and Tobago Medical Association was informed, regarding an outbreak in Santo Domingo, by Dr Matthew Beaubrun, of the Medical Association of Jamaica, who requested a donation of vaccine from Trinidad. At a meeting of the TTMA executive, when the correspondence was read, the Secretary was asked to notify the Government's Ministry of Health of this information and to offer the assistance of the TTMA in whatever measures the Ministry deemed fit.

Following the previous epidemic, an inoculation campaign was instituted by the Ministry, but all statistics pointed to the fact that, despite this, there was a tremendous and epidemiologically dangerous percentage of the population, especially between the ages of 0-5 years, who were susceptible.

Despite all the above, there is no indication that the Government took any substantial steps, until November 1971, to alert the population to the impending danger and/or immunise the population.

Late in 1971, several proved cases appeared, and with the announcement of deaths, the population appeared suddenly to have become alert to the danger and started presenting themselves in large numbers for the vaccine at Health Centres and Private Practitioners' offices.

There are reports of large batches of vaccines being allowed to thaw out at room temperature, twenty-four hours before use at certain centres, and certain private practitioners report that on some occasions their supplies from private firms in Port of Spain arrived at their offices at van temperature.

As the epidemic receded, only a small proportion of persons presented their children for the second and third doses and very few adults returned for their second doses.

The official pronouncement of the Ministry of Health (through Dr Siung, Principal Medical Officer of Health) is that this has been just another epidemic of poliomyelitis, that we have had worse epidemics in the past, and that there has been too much publicity – even panic – in the local press.

Private practitioners have been accused in the press of profiteering from the epidemic, and charging up to $5 for each oral dose of the vaccine.

Government has issued the statement that in future no child will be admitted to school (at age five years or more) without documentary evidence of vaccination against poliomyelitis.

Discussion

There is no controversy, in the light of the above findings, that the epidemic in Trinidad and Tobago was entirely unnecessary, in the sense that if the early warnings had been heeded by the authorities and early vaccination – a completely feasible project – had been instituted by June 1971, there would have been no epidemic.

It is important that we should discover the exact reasons and location of breakdown in the chain of information and execution of policy which was responsible for the epidemic. In this day and age, it is not enough to adopt the attitude that such things are in the nature of unavoidable misfortunes, 'acts of God' so to speak. It would also be fatal for many of the future generations if we were to say to ourselves, "Well, this has already happened, why dig up the muck of the past." In our profession, we have learned that accurate post mortem examinations are not only an indispensable aid to diagnosis in some instances, but that examinations done routinely have proved to be invaluable in determining prophylaxis and treatment. It is in this spirit that the present discussion and recommendations are made.

Sociological and Psychological Considerations

Unlike most developed countries, especially those with a long history of democratic institutions, Trinidad and Tobago is characterised by having a population which responds more to compulsion than to education and persuasion. In general also, the people of this country are inclined to postpone medical treatment until the danger of death is apparent, or until severe pain or discomfort 'forces' them to do so. Again, as soon as the immediate pain or fatal threat has been alleviated, the patient generally returns with extreme reluctance (if at all) for further treatment, no matter how strongly the practitioner may have stressed its importance.

Prophylaxis by persuasion and education is well nigh impossible in these conditions. This is not to say that long term educational measures are not important, indeed, vital to the development of our country. We know that there is a considerable number of people who have gained sufficient insight into this problem, to appreciate the role that slavery and indenture followed by a long period of paternalism and political dependence play in the persistence of these social attitudes to health and hygiene. Here, there is a role for village council, county council and so on. It must be recognised that immunisation by invitation alone cannot be expected to work in this country for at least another ten years.

Government's decision not to admit children to school without proof of certain immunisations (including polio) does not go far enough. It is easily predictable that there will be a mad rush on the part of parents to give their children their *first* shots on the eve of application for entrance to school, so there will still be a huge non-resistant group between the ages of 0-5 years.

The solution seems to be to provide legislation making immunisation compulsory (as in the case of smallpox), starting before, say, the age of five months. A schedule should be provided to the mother of each child as soon as the birth is registered. This card would be a guide for immunisations and should be in permanent form, to last a lifetime.

It follows, that all vaccines should be available free of charge at all health offices and centres. The possibility of supplying vaccines to private practitioners free of charge should also be considered, but this would be an attempt to deal piecemeal with the question of comprehensive medical care involving the private sector which does in fact form part of the proposals of another sub-committee of the TTMA. This proposal will be referred to again in this report in another context.

Ethical Considerations

It is the usual practice in this country to search for and publicise the role of scapegoats when a tragedy has occurred. This is sometimes done to divert attention from the real causes. In the recent poliomyelitis epidemic, private practitioners were accused of profiteering, that is, charging up to $5 for a single oral dose of vaccine. Private investigations indeed reveal that some doctors did so, but the more usual charge was $2 and $3. After considering the possible wastage, I find that charges of up to $3 were reasonable, especially in view of the fact that vaccines were available free at government centres if persons wished to take it there. Charges of profiteering would certainly be of some substance if private practitioners were the only ones who possessed the vaccine, and people were compelled by circumstances to pay for the shot. The real failure was that, because of delay, there was a mad rush at the government centres, resulting in a certain degree of queuing for the shot, so people whose time was more valuable than the private doctors' fees, voluntarily sought such attention. Again, the beneficial role of a full, comprehensive, pre-paid scheme would be seen to advantage in obviating panic crowds at health centres.

The shipping and storage of vaccines, both for use at centres and by private practitioners, during the last epidemic needs to be further investigated. There is evidence that refrigeration standards were not observed.

Administrative and Political

This committee is unable to understand why the warnings of Dr Ardoin were not acted upon until, at the latest, June 1971. It is important to pinpoint the exact link in the chain of information/execution which broke before the epidemic. Until this is discovered, there is likely to be much conjecture as to the point of failure.

Already, it is suggested that the Cabinet was so involved in pre-election and post-election politics, at the crucial stages of the spread of the wild virus, that the warnings of the technical officers were ignored. This is a matter which ought to be investigated, and this committee recommends that a letter be forwarded to the Minister of Health asking for a report of what happened as from the time of Dr Ardoin's warnings: more particularly, to whom was the warning given, and what action was taken.

Whether or not breakdown had occurred at the political level, this unfortunate sequence of events gives strong support to the view that the entire question of the health care of the population should be reviewed and re-organised, and underlines the importance of the recommendations of the TTMA sub-committee, concerned that a full comprehensive pre-paid health corporation, run by a statutory board answerable directly to parliament and politically uninvolved in its day to day operations, should take over from Government in the very near future.

(Report submitted on 15th April, 1972)

ADDENDUM: 18.5.72: Recent cases (this week) are reported to have had one or two doses of vaccine: it is possible that faulty vaccine could have contributed to the persistence of susceptibility.

ADDENDUM: 15.9.94: Shortly after this report was published, an excellent Record of Immunisation card with comprehensive recommendations printed on it was produced by our Ministry of Health and supplied to all health centres and to private practitioners who requested it.

Welcome to Tobago, Doctors

(Welcoming address at International Medical Convention, October 17th to 19th, 1975)

As President of the Trinidad and Tobago Medical Association, I have great pleasure in welcoming you to the first ever International Medical Convention to be held in this country. I have a special word of welcome for returning prodigal sons and daughters: unlike the biblical wanderer you have come back with your assets multiplied rather than exhausted. Participating doctors will be giving us the benefit of their work in all parts of the world. There is no doubt that your contributions will be invaluable in their own right. But, there may be some practical difficulty in making use of your findings and recommendations in the milieu of another and somewhat different country – for a variety of reasons. Sometimes the receptivity of the soil may not do justice to the genetic merit of the seed, even the seed which you, my esteemed colleagues will sow this weekend in generous abundance. For this reason, therefore, may I be permitted to relate a few facts and figures which may be relevant at the eventual discussion of your papers.

Both our islands together have an area of about two thousand square miles. Our contiguous continental shelf, over which we have jurisdiction, adds another ten thousand square miles. For a developing country, we have a very high per capita income, namely TT$3,000. We should compare this with Ghana: $1,000, the Philippines: $500, India: $250, Sri Lanka: $50. We should also contrast these figures with those of some highly developed nations, for example the United Kingdom: $7,000, Canada: $11,000 and the USA: $12,000. These figures are all in Trinidad and Tobago dollars.

Now, the $3,000 for Trinidad and Tobago multiplied by our million people gives a national income of three billion dollars. Our annual budget, by comparison, is one billion dollars. The indications are, therefore, that for a small nation our annual accumulation of reserves, due at present largely to our petroleum exports and held largely in US dollars is quite fantastic.

How is this income earned by our population? Here are some average figures: 20% of the population earn 80% of the income and 80% earn 20%. Doctors tend to gravitate towards the first bracket! But 50% of the households receive less than $1,000 per annum. We have seventy thousand unemployed, or 15% of our work force. These people have no unemployment benefits.

In other words, half of our population are living below the poverty line, and this is an extremely important fact with reference to health care. Quite apart from the factors of malnutrition and poor sanitation inherent in conditions of poverty, poor people cannot pay doctors' and pharmacists' bills.

In Trinidad and Tobago, private medical and surgical practice – both general and specialist – exist side by side with a free government service available to all. The private fee, payable by the patient, exclusive of drugs and surgery, varies from $3 to $25, with an average at about $10. The average payment to the government doctor, based on the number of patients attended to and on salaries and emoluments, works out at thirty three cents per patient! While there is considerable overlap, both at doctor and patient level, the government service caters largely to the 50% of the population below the poverty line of $1,000.

The constant migration of doctors from the government service into private practice is, therefore, easy to understand. So, also, is the physical and emotional strain on the residual task force, and the constant jeopardy of the doctor-patient relationship in the government health services.

During the course of this convention, you will hear something of the medical, surgical and pathological problems of this country. One of these is protein calorie deficiency especially in young infants, caused by the inability of mothers to afford the price of milk, which is largely imported.

The TTMA (as we affectionately refer to our association) made representations to government on this subject about one year ago, and our efforts culminated with a statement in the press (August 31st, 1975) by the President. We are happy to note that two weeks ago the import duty on baby feeds was considerably reduced, thus enabling mothers to buy milk for their babies and to drink more themselves to produce more human breast milk.

The TTMA now proposes to submit concrete proposals for the more permanent solution, viz. proposals for the more extensive and less expensive production of milk and milk equivalents on Trinidad and Tobago farms.

In endocrinological terms: we in the TTMA are beginning to understand the complex interplay of clinical, journalistic, ministerial and fiscal hormones which produce lactation in the sacred cow. Remember, the word 'hormone' is derived from the Greek, meaning a 'Kissinger' – I beg your pardon, a 'messenger'.

From the medical standpoint, local agricultural production of food is of paramount importance. We import $150 million worth of foodstuffs and animal feeds each year, including milk and milk products, corn and soya beans and their products, fish and fish products and, paradoxically, cocoa and sugar products!

We also have two hundred thousand acres of fertile arable lands, reclaimed by bush for such a long time that they have achieved the remarkable status of secondary virginity hoping for a second spring! As indices of our food production potential – without in any way restricting the number of food crop species to be used – let us consider that these acres can produce six hundred million pounds of corn and three hundred million pounds of soya beans, worth together $180 million per annum or $30 million more than our food import bill!

As you know, our land is cultivable for twelve months each year. The direct effect of production of agricultural raw materials, plus the multiplier effect of daughter industries based on them, could easily add another $1,000 to our per capita income.

But what is more important, from the medical standpoint, is that such increased human activity would considerably reduce nutritional and other debilitating disease, psychological problems and the incidence of crime, including crimes of violence, all of which now present a crushing burden on our health services.

Again, on the subject of protein starvation: our fishermen on the south coast of Trinidad are today dumping approximately twenty thousand pounds in weight of first class fresh fish per day, for want of cold storage facilities. This occurs during the months of September and October each year. They sell what they can at twenty cents per pound. Yet we import salted cod at $1.50 per pound, and tinned salmon at $3.50 per pound from Canada.

It is no wonder that the per capita income of the Canadians is $11,000, and that they have a full comprehensive health plan with a lucrative fee for service, not our paltry thirty three cents per patient – and that the medical brain drain flows, with Gulf Stream persistence, from the West Indies to Canada and the USA.

Incidentally, I am sure that our Venezuelan colleagues present here today must be sorry to hear of the wastage of the Cavali and Carite fish which have come to us from their Orinoco estuary, twelve miles away – of their own free will and accord, without benefit of protocol.

Canada is now limiting the influx of West Indian doctors; of course, she must protect her own medical market. Charity – if I may thus euphemistically refer to their fee for service – begins at home! Yet, as an international gathering – and I trust that we present here today regard ourselves not as an aggregation of national representatives, but as a congregation of international doctors serving mankind as a whole – let this international congregation realise that this is by no means the final solution of the question. (The resemblance to Nazi terminology may not be entirely coincidental). We must appreciate that the reason our doctors seek a living in metropolitan countries lies basically with the pathetic underdevelopment of our superabundant resources.

It is at this basic level that United Nations agencies could cooperate with us even more intensively, so that one inevitable result would be the reversal of the brain drain to the snows of increasingly more frigid nations from the salubrious climate of Trinidad and Tobago. We do not spurn the intensive care unit, but we welcome with enthusiasm the tractor, the trawler, the plough.

I trust, my dear colleagues, my friends, that I have been able – however briefly and sketchily – to indicate some of the synapses, to portray the unity of medicine, society, economics and even international affairs. Against this background, let us measure our efforts this weekend.

I trust that when – say, in five years time – another convention is held in this island, a future president will be able to affirm that what, I am sure, we all yearn for today has, in fact, taken place, and that we are fully ready to participate in the explosion of scientific achievement that a sneak preview of the titles of your papers promises at this convention.

In conclusion, my dear friends, may I express the hope that you will find the warmth and variety of form and colour of these surroundings reflected in our temperament and in our souls. As citizens of Trinidad and Tobago, we trust that your stay in Tobago – by far the most unspoilt and most beautiful part of our country – will enable you to share in all the natural virtues which we may have to offer

Enjoy yourselves: let your pleasure be unrestrained.

Impotence

Of the one hundred young men and boys who consult me because they fail to get an erection when the occasion demands, only one or two have some diagnosable condition which could have contributed to such malfunction – usually diabetes or the use of some drug. The reason for their impotence has, in the vast majority of cases, been psychological. Of men over sixty, three quarters have firm, reasonably sized testicles which I interpret to mean that they are producing a proper supply of male hormones. Most of these also have no trace of organic disease, but a definite history of anxiety, depression and domestic, financial or other tension at their work. To these, I offer psychological advice, after telling them the following true story.

When I was a student at McGill University in 1942, a close friend of mine had a charming, petite Canadian girlfriend with whom he had been having intimate relations, two or three times per week, for over six months. She lived on the same street – University Street about ten houses away. One day, after his lunch, on his way to his Bacteriology class, he dropped in to see her, and after a few ardent, if hurried, caresses, he attempted intercourse. Alas, his organ would not respond. Devastated and utterly disconsolate at its stubborn limpness, he sadly dressed, picked up his microscope, looked at his wristwatch and noted that he had just ten minutes to arrive at the laboratory. His next twenty-four hours were sheer mental agony and depression: was he impotent? Would he be like this for the rest of his life?

The following day the telephone rang. It was his girlfriend. She wanted to see him. "But don't come at lunchtime," she requested, "Come after classes when you have nothing else to do."

That evening, she was as kind and as wise as she was physically attractive. "There is nothing wrong with you," she told him, "Yesterday you were in too much of a hurry: your mind was on your watch and on the clock in the Bacteriology lab while it should have been here," as she passed her hand gently over her lower abdomen.

Fifty-two years have passed since my friend learned this lesson about himself. He continues to be a very sensitive soul, and has had temporary bouts of impotence from time to time, but these have never kept him down: he has had two wives, more than half a dozen children and several grandchildren. He enjoys sexual intercourse now – at the age of over seventy – on an average of three times a week, to the complete orgasmic satisfaction of his spouse and himself!

Libido

Men over sixty and women over fifty commonly seek my advice regarding their loss of sexual drive – their libido. These are couples who have been living together for decades, often married by parental arrangement in their early teens, and who have several children and grandchildren with no financial, domestic or pathological problems, and obviously very much in love. They each feel that they are doing their partner a disservice by chronically not being 'in the mood'. Very often, the wife suspects infidelity and occasionally her suspicions are justifiable.

It is obviously often the case that they are just too accustomed to each other and have developed a 'brother-sister' relationship, but I have discovered that in most instances a dry introitus is an extremely potent deterrent to a man's libido, a common source of friction, and an encouragement for him to slip – as it were – into infidelity. Muslim men, who utilise their religion's acceptance of polygamy and marry younger wives in turn (Islam permits four), do not appear to lose their libido. This is one of the many pragmatic tenets of Islamic culture.

I generally recommend a lubricating jelly, which the wife may use without her partner's knowledge if necessary. The patented 'K-Y Gel' is cheap and effective, but my recommended preference is an oestrogen cream such as 'Premarin'. This costs about $70 Trinidad and Tobago currency (about eleven US dollars or eight pounds sterling.) One tube has enough for about twenty occasions and three and a half TT dollars is a small price to pay for each happy communion in the lives of these dear couples.

Dozens of satisfied ladies and gentlemen have returned to thank me for such advice. Oestrogen creams have the added advantage of improving the vaginal and vulval linings, and alleviating some of their defects. It appears that portions of the hormones in the cream are absorbed into the bloodstream, resulting in the general well-being of these ladies, and by extension, in the happiness of their partners.

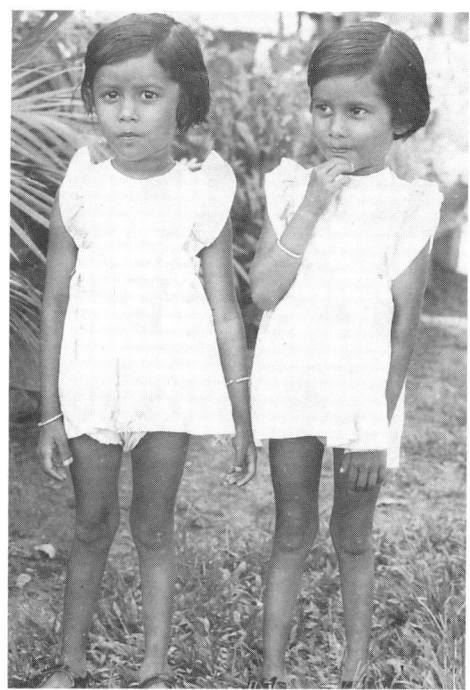

Annabelle and Christabelle. Note Annabelle's right thumb.

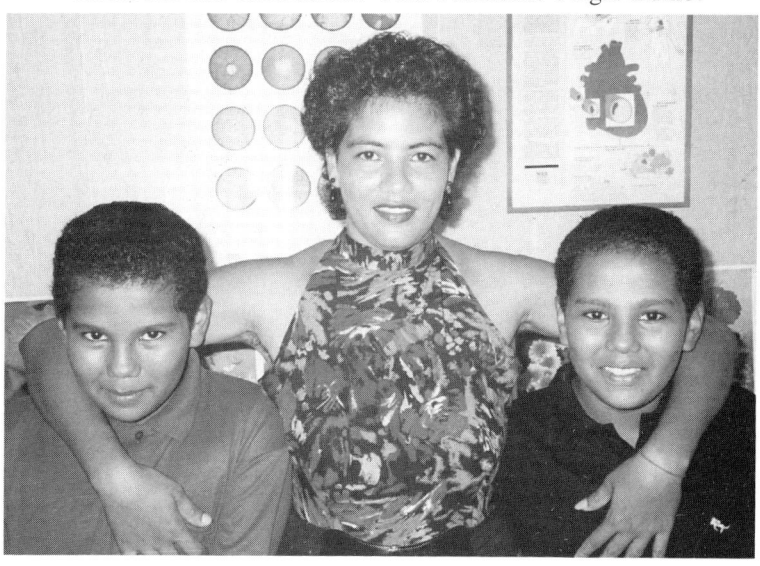

Identical twins, Vince and Vincent at age twelve with their mother.
Their ancestry includes persons of Spanish, East Indian, Chinese,
African and Scottish origin.
Vince is more reserved and excels in mathematics. Vincent is
extrovert and excels in literature.

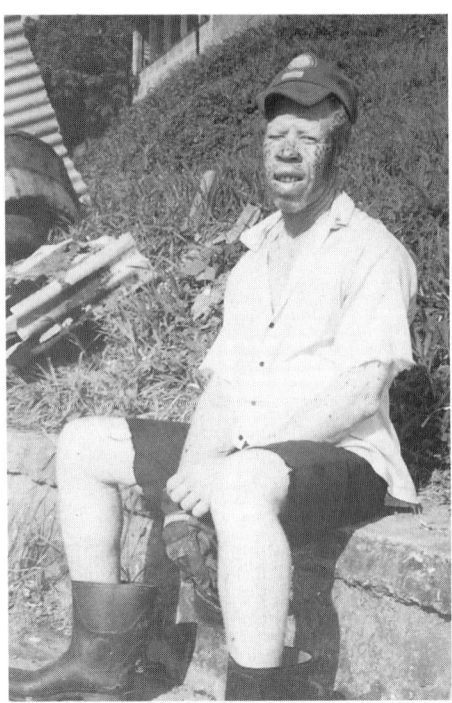

Adult Albino – Afro-Trinidadian.

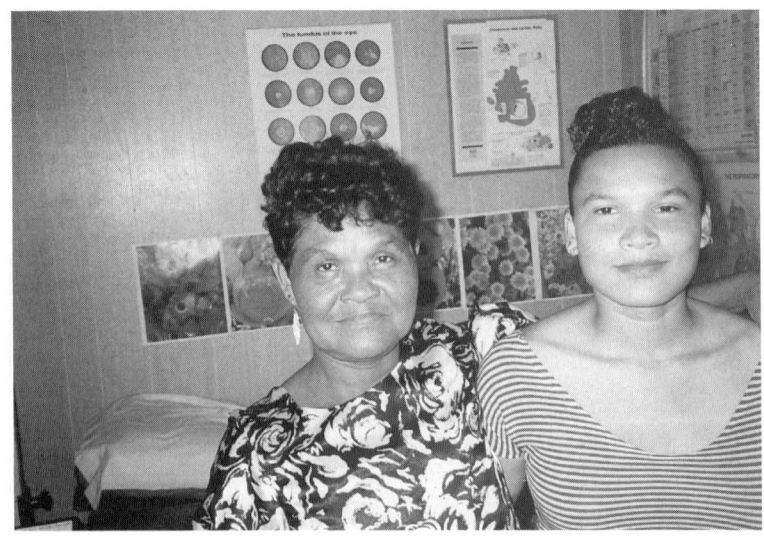

Half-Carib and half-Spanish mother. Father had the same ancestry. The daughter appears to have received more Spanish than Carib genes.

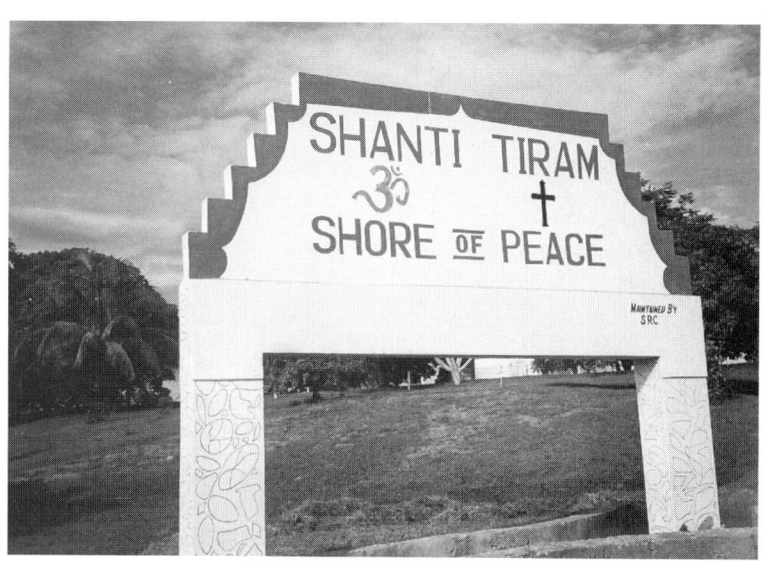

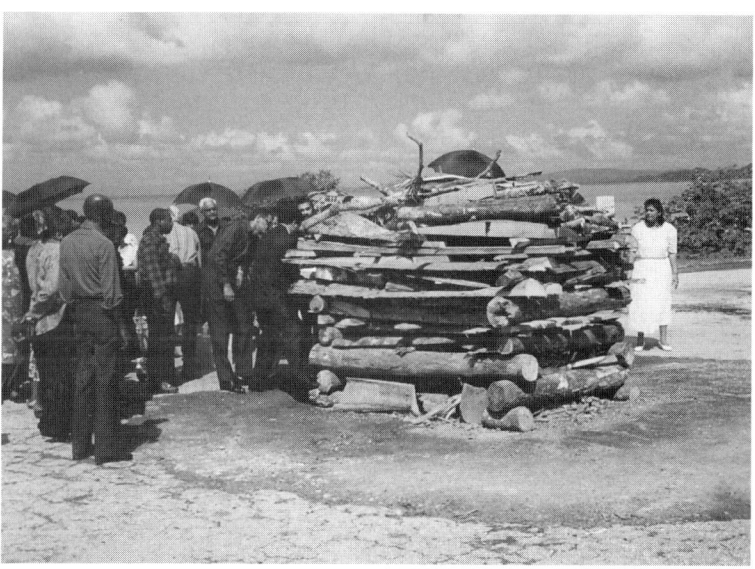

Body being inserted into pyre.

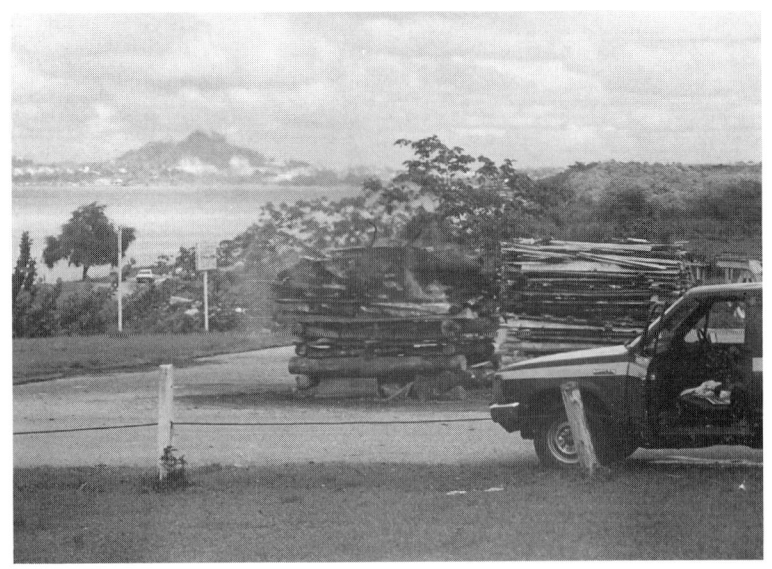

Start of combustion.

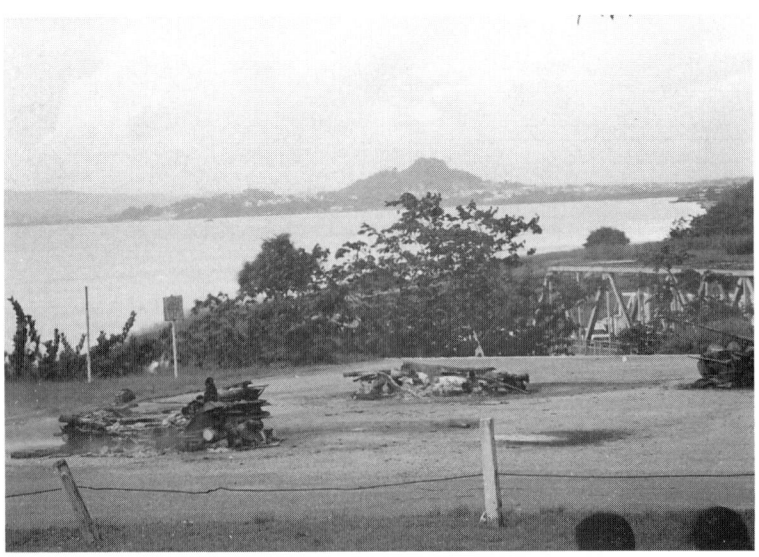

Near the end of combustion. Godineau Bridge and Gulf of Paria in the middle ground. City of San Fernando and Naparima Hill in the background.

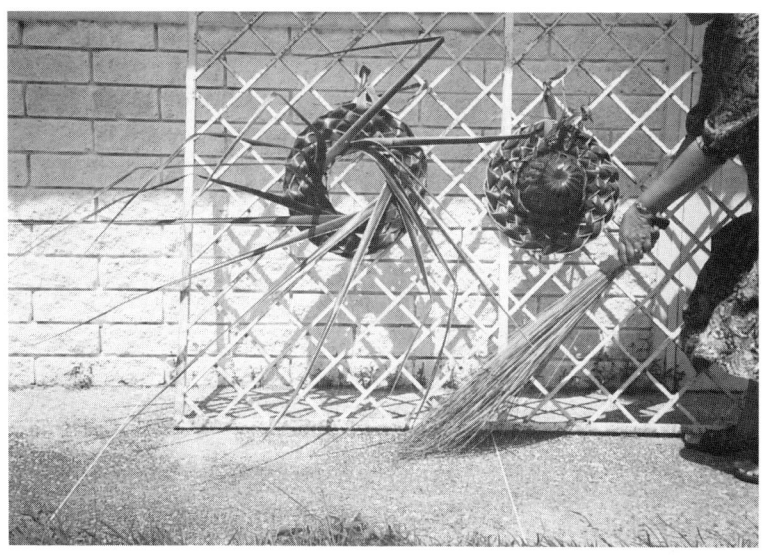

The versatile coconut leaf. *Left:* Start of a hat. *Right:* The finished product. *In front:* The Cocoyea broom.

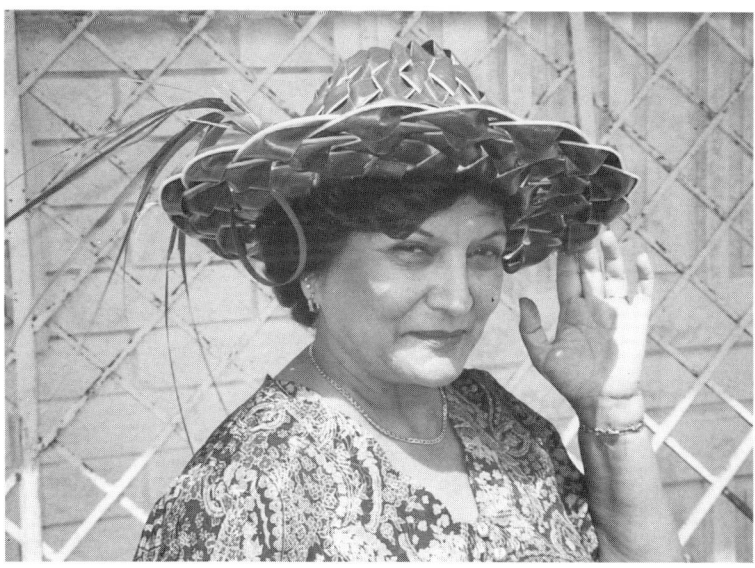

A 'Rebirth House' trainee can make this hat in ninety minutes. Tourists pay $10 for it.

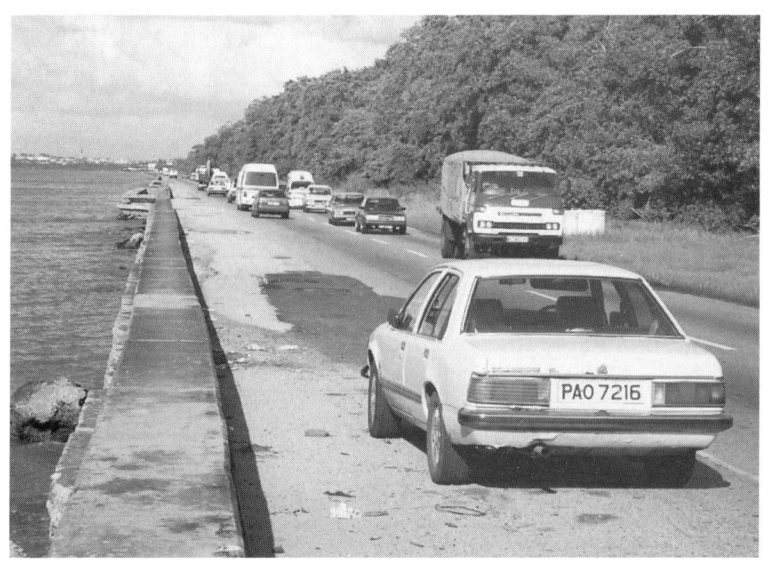

Mosquito Creek Road, now polluted by heavy traffic.

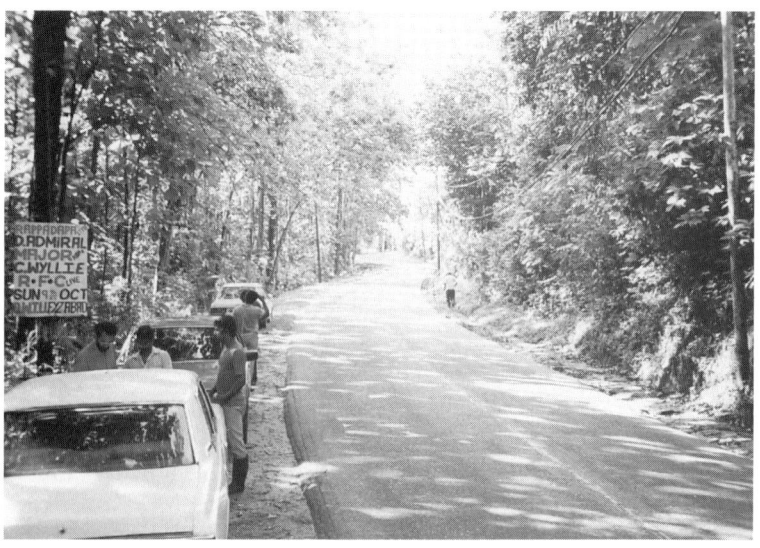

Papa Pierre Forest Road, formerly an oxygen-rich drive.

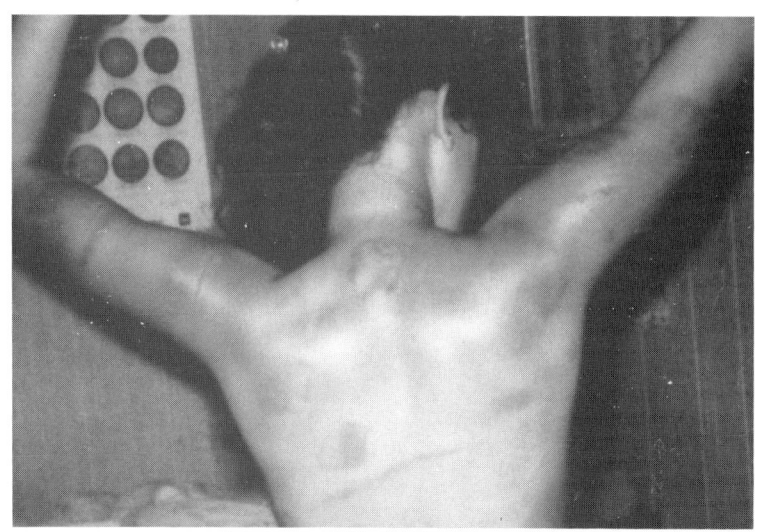

After 'Planass' attack.

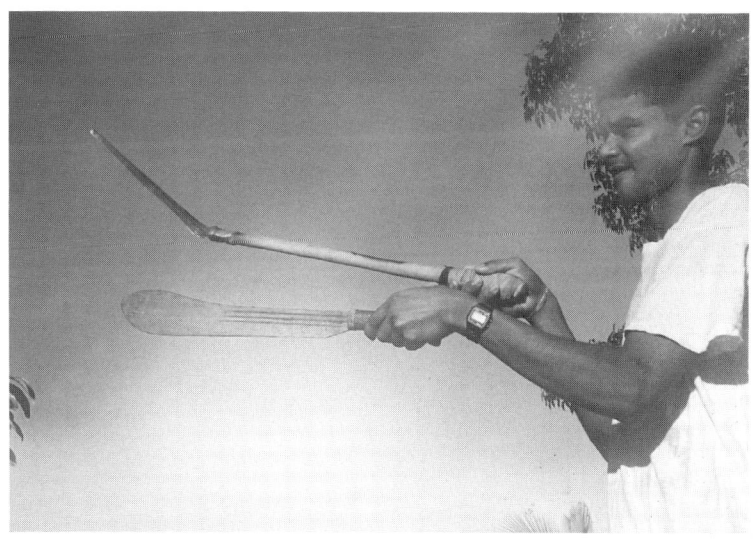

Top instrument: 'Brushing' cutlass used for cutting grass.
The narrow blade was used with 'moderate force' to penetrate
the rib cage and heart of victim referred to under 'Anatomical
Concepts'.
Lower instrument: Regular cutlass suitable for 'planassing'.

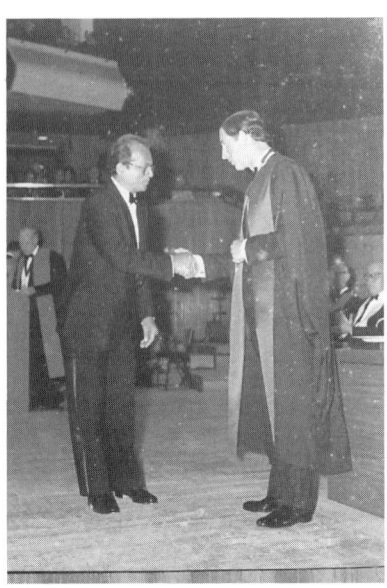

Author meets Prince Charles, president of British Medical
Association, at London conference.
Photograph by Official Conference Photographer

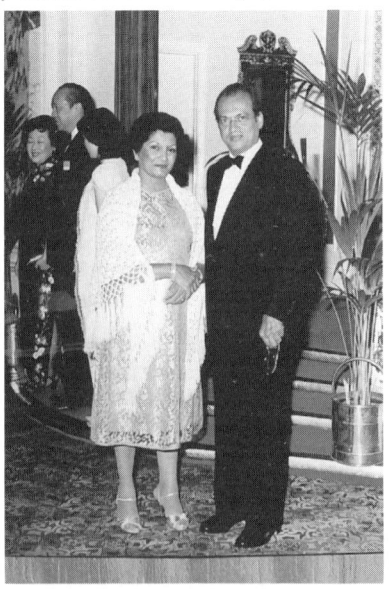

The author and spouse at BMA conference, London.
Photograph by Official Conference Photographer

'Tropical Oils' and Cholesterol

The current fears of an elevated cholesterol in the blood – especially of low density lipo-proteins – have reached Trinidad and Tobago. These fears are obscenely capitalised upon by some of our cooking oil manufacturers who label their wares, 'Contains No Cholesterol'. Now most educated people know that vegetable oils do not contain cholesterol. Plants do not make this stuff, animals do. The danger is in the consumption of animal products loaded with cholesterol and with saturated fats.

Then there are the manufacturers of corn and soya bean oil who, in metropolitan countries, by intensive lobbying in their media, repeatedly castigate so-called 'Tropical Oils' as conducive to cholesterol formation. Indeed, both corn (maize) and soya beans are grown in the tropics and can produce oil for consumption, but the primary target of these unscrupulous advertisers is coconut oil – a powerful competitor for the cooking oil market.

Coconut oil has been consumed by tropical people all over the globe for countless generations, and no pathologist has yet found that these individuals have a higher cholesterol level or more hardening of the arteries by atherosclerosis than their temperate counterparts. Perhaps their judicious consumption of fish oils, and the relative absence of mammalian fats in their diets, combined with a much less stressful lifestyle, are the reasons for their comparative vascular health.

It is tragic that in order to discredit an economic competitor, such immoral insinuations should be employed, especially when the export of coconut products is such an important source of foreign exchange for so many tropical nations. The degree of unsaturation of oils is generally determined from the 'iodine value' and the following list is instructive:

Source	Iodine Value	Source	Iodine Value
Soyabean	130-150	Sardine	170-190
Corn (Maize)	124-140	Herring	120-145
Sunflower	120-140	Cod liver	120-180
Peanut	85-100	Coconut	8-10
Olive oil	75-95	Butter	25-40

Evidently, a combination in the diet of coconut oil and fish oils, or coconut and sunflower oil, in suitable proportions would satisfy both the fat calorie requirements and the polyunsaturated fat needs of an individual.

In many parts of the tropics, sunflower will grow like a weed, and perhaps its cultivation should be encouraged on an economic scale in order to provide an additive to commercially marketed coconut oil.

A Doctor and His Car

A doctor is supposed to have a private car, and use it at all times. When I lived in Siparia – a quarter of a mile away from my office – it was very useful to be able to arrive at work in three minutes, in any kind of weather. On fine days, I often strolled across the extensive Siparia savannah, after lunch, back to the office. I was invariably asked many times on these trips, "Doctor, what happen to your car?" Once, while taking an afternoon stroll with six of my children around the block, I was offered a lift no fewer than three times by my patients! In Trinidad and Tobago, a car is not only a necessity but also a potent status symbol. For me, it has always been merely an extension of my legs. I kept my first car, the Hillman Minx, for ten years. They made good cars in those days, and good car parts and accessories. During those years of extremely rigorous use, I never needed to change the storage battery, and I simply recapped the worn tyres. When I bought my second car – a 1952 model De Soto – second hand to boot, I kept the Hillman, since it consumed less gasoline, and used the De Soto for special social occasions. I kept the De Soto for twelve years, and finally, when I bought another car, I gave her to Mr Bruce, the mechanic who looked after her, to be used as spare parts.

My patients forever asked me, "Doctor, why don't you buy a Jaguar like Dr P or a Mercedes like Dr M?" They could never believe that I was not in the status symbol race.

In Siparia, my home and my office were at opposite ends of the same block, which had a perimeter of half a mile so that the trip from home to office and vice versa could be done either in a clockwise or a anticlockwise direction with the same result in time and mileage. My practice was to approach my office from the east in the morning, so that, when I parked alongside my office, the morning to midday sun was at the back of the parked car. After lunch, I did the opposite, so that the midday to evening sun did not enter through the front windshield. Because of the locations of my home and office, described above, it was always unnecessary to turn my car around – I just drove off and took the way home in the direction in which the car was facing.

Now you can understand what I am about to relate: the above system after twenty-five years, had become automatic and so, about a week after my family and I moved to La Romaine, having sold our Siparia home to Mr Boodram, a school teacher, I got into my car after work and drove down High Street, turned into Oropouche Road, and instead of continuing on this road towards La Romaine, I turned into Gambal Street, into my old driveway, into my old garage, switched off my engine, got out of the car, and as I was about to take up my bag and close the door, I saw a strange woman standing on the threshold! Only then did I realise that I was in the wrong place. I hid my embarrassment, however, by saying to Mrs Boodram, "I just came to see how you and your family are settling in. And how is Penny getting on?" (Penny was a female deer which I had left for the Boodrams at their request. She was one of fourteen brockets – our indigenous wild deer – which I was rearing. I took the other thirteen with me to La Romaine. Penny was born at the time one of our ladies – Miss Penny Commissiong – won the Miss Universe beauty contest).

My driving by reflex – indeed a form of automatism – is very relaxing. The higher centres of my brain have solved many distant problems and formulated many plans while the lower centres were dodging the mundane traffic on the roads, but this dichotomy twice got me involved in accidents. On both occasions, while I was working out political plans, motor vehicles passed me, at fifty miles an hour to my forty, and stopped suddenly in front of me to avoid hitting the vehicle which I was complacently following. On both occasions, my car skidded in response to my slamming on the foot brakes, but only stopped on impact. I should have anticipated the manoeuvre of the driver behind me, but while my body was driving, my mind was elsewhere.

I enjoy driving to and from work on the familiar twenty kilometres of coastal, small village and forest road. But how I wish that we already had electric cars on the roads instead of the foully polluting machines now in existence. The three-mile coastal road – the so-called Mosquito Creek – used to be a wonderfully invigorating journey when motor cars were few, but today, even with a strong sea breeze blowing, the acrid smell of nitrogen and sulphur oxides and the soot from partly burned fuel are occasionally exhausting.

I remember how pleasantly we traversed the one-mile road which wound its way through the forest reserve approaching Siparia. The air used to be cool and fresh. My first recollection of this particular stretch was of driving through on a buggy drawn by a horse called 'Steplight', with my maternal grandfather. I must have been three years old at the time. Later, I made this trip with my uncle in his model-T Ford. Having traversed this route a thousand times since then, every curve, every cliff, every wayside boulder has become familiar to me. For many decades, there used to be a huge sandstone boulder alongside this road, part of the parent rock exposed during the excavation for laying down the track for the roadway. This rock gave the name for the entire forested area: 'Papa Pierre'. Alas, today the stench of the gasoline engine permeates this once pristine retreat. In our islands, it is seldom necessary to travel faster than the legal speed limit of fifty miles an hour on open roads and thirty miles through built up areas. Yet we import and drive cars which are manufactured to go at speeds of one hundred and twenty man hour! What a waste! Perhaps even in my lifetime, our politicians and our businessmen and our consumers will come to their senses and ensure that most gasoline and diesel consuming vehicles are replaced by non-polluting electric ones.

The Role of the General Practitioner in Providing Primary Care

Paper presented to the Caribbean Medical Conference.
(Reprinted from the CMJ *Vol 38 No 1. 1977)*

After some consideration of the topic allocated to me, it seemed that the greatest danger inherent in my task was that, with a superfluity of professionalism, I might be carried away to describe the functioning of the practitioner, number of patients, society, secondary care and governments in ideal terms such as I should like them to be. This appears to be the image portrayed for television viewers by productions, like *Dr Kildare*, *Marcus Welby*, *Medical Centre* and so on, which stimulate the desires of citizens in a Caribbean where most things are very far from ideal. It is no wonder that the Caribbean citizen is more and more outraged, when the realities of primary and secondary care fall below his television-inspired expectations.

A more rewarding course seemed to me to describe the situation, as it has existed in Trinidad and Tobago during the past five years (1971 to 1976), stressing at the outset that existing conditions were not invented *de novo* in 1971, but are a natural evolution of forces at work before Columbus through Chacon, Abercromby, slavery, indenture, the Colonial Office, and finally Whitehall and political independence.

Most of what I will describe is based on my experience in Siparia and San Fernando, Trinidad. There will doubtless be close similarities in the other rural and semi-rural parts of the Caribbean, and there will be marked differences with many of the more urban areas. These differences will probably be more in degree, and in shift of balance, rather than in basic quality, and I trust, therefore, that in attempting to correct our deficiencies – which is the main purpose of my approach – this paper will, in some small measure, assist doctors and Governments, present and future, in all Caribbean countries from 1976 onwards.

Social Factors

By definition of 'Primary Care', the GP is the first 'practitioner' who is consulted by anyone who has reason to believe that he or she may not be in good health. In practice this is not always so: we still have numerous obeah men who treat anaemia, depression, schizophrenia, tabanca and so on. These do little harm. However, we have local midwives who treat amenorrhoea quite drastically, and pundits who attempt to jharray or charm bile pigments away from cases of jaundice, wheezing from asthma patients and scorpion venom from young and old.

In all fairness to the sophistication of the modern patient, we must state that this diversion of primary care is usually little more than just that, a preliminary diversion, in order to pander to the wishes of older relatives, and the patient soon finds his or her way to the GP, not when the cause of the amenorrhoea is visually obvious or the haemorrhage too severe, or the skin more icteric, or the asthmatic cyanotic or the scorpion-stung subject collapsed and vomiting, but well within the hour. Patients today do appreciate the value of the GP in his role as primary attendant for all illnesses.

Yet, we do see many patients *in proxime extremis*: gross anaemia from parasites, iron deficiency, avitaminosis and hypoproteinaemia, exsanguination from amateur abortion, cardiac failure from scorpion stings and other serious illnesses. These are not the result of ignorance, social custom or the geographical unavailability of the GP. Nearly all of these patients are poor.

Economic Factors

In theory, there is a twenty-four hour, free, GP medical service run by the Ministry of Health. This is the District Medical Officer system, inherited from colonial times when in most rural areas he was the only doctor in his extensive district. He lived in the biggest town or village in the area, in government quarters, and attended up to seven health offices, for two hours, each week. He was on call twenty-four hours per day, he was also the police surgeon, and viewed dead bodies, and did post mortem dissections when required. He received a monthly salary, plus certain per-service fees, civil service travelling allowances, a duty free car, and he was also allowed unfettered private practice for private fees.

Today, very few DMOs live in their government quarters or even in their districts, many of them do not visit their health offices for weeks. Very often, they are not available for police cases, and even for viewing dead bodies. The result is that a great deal of this work is thrust upon the purely private practitioners of the districts. It is, of course, always embarrassing for an unsubsidised private doctor to be approached by an impecunious, poor, injured or seriously ill patient and asked for credit, which in practice usually means free treatment. GPs may be excused for doing this service somewhat grudgingly when they think of the taxes they pay to subsidise DMOs who are not there when required.

Yet the fault is not with the individuals who hold the posts. The DMO system is anachronistic to the point of obsolescence. The populations of the districts have grown, and the isolation has disappeared to the point where the very idea of a *District* Medical Officer is ridiculous. There is nothing that a DMO does or can do that another GP is not also doing or can do just as efficiently.

The *raisons d'être* of the DMO are isolation, poverty and the unavailability of a doctor. In practice, his appointment does not solve the poverty problem – which is just as accentuated today as it was twenty years ago; isolation is not a factor; and the question of a doctor not being available is not caused by deficient supply, because the patient can usually get several of them, including the DMO, at their private offices between nine in the morning and four in the afternoon on non-holiday weekdays. It is a question of proper motivation and the efficient utilisation of our adequate resources by proper organisation.

Infrastructure

The infrastructures needed by citizens in general and by industries and business include roads, water supply, electricity, telephone, police service and so on. In addition to these, there are certain infrastructures for general practice which must be there, even though they are used only intermittently by the doctor. These include, X-ray and laboratory facilities, ambulance service and the availability of secondary care.

Now, inefficiency and breakdowns in general infrastructures occur as a result of overloading of unexpanded facilities for example traffic jams, road accidents, electricity load shedding (I am typing this after waiting for twelve hours without electricity on Easter Monday – I wonder what happened to my vaccines?) dry taps, somebody else's conversation on the telephone or none at all.

In medicine, a patient, for the same reason, may have to wait two months for an IVP or a cholecystogram, and three to four months for a barium meal. He would get them privately within seven days. The private roads are not so congested, if you can pay the toll!

By contrast, pathological investigations are prompt. They are not so popular as X-rays. The greatest delay in these cases is another infrastructure – the post office. It takes an average of seven days to cover fifteen miles, and ten days to cover fifty miles. Naturally, we rely heavily on smell to differentiate GC from syphilis. I know a DMO who travels to collect his reports, and charges travelling mileage for the trip – $15 per trip; but, as I have said, the discordance is not of the singer, but of the song.

If a GP waited for an ambulance to send all his severely ill patients to hospital, he would be issuing many more death certificates. Thank God for our very efficient PH taxi service! The regular taximen say they (private cars working as taxis) have been prostituted and would have them prosecuted, and persecuted, but patients whose lives have been saved by them when they could not get an ambulance, say they should be proliferated and doubly remunerated.

The average waiting time for routine non-acute specialist consultation at the San Fernando General Hospital varies from one to three months. The same doctor will see the same patient privately within seven days. A case of hernia, while waiting to have his repair after a twelve month appointment at the Outpatients' Clinic, will have it done by the same doctor privately within a week.

Some unscrupulous doctors will accept donations from patients who wish to have operations done quickly in a government hospital. Paradoxically, the GP often has the greatest difficulty in persuading certain very seriously ill patients to go to hospital. They say they are not looked after properly, not medically, but that the nursing care is as near to absent as possible, the food is bad, bed sheets and toilets are dirty, nurses are rude and heartless. There is no doubt that some of these reports are exaggerated, but at the same time, it is true that most of the nurses are not happy in their work. By contrast, there are very few complaints about conditions at our larger, private, nursing homes.

Medico-Legal Affairs

General Medical Practitioners are often called upon to examine patients associated with the alleged committing of crime. There is usually little difficulty in these matters when the police have summoned the doctor as witness for the prosecution. The police, counsel – especially for the prosecution – and the magistrate are usually very considerate and show the utmost respect for the doctor's report, opinion and time. But, it is usually the opposite when the doctor appears for one who complains that he was beaten by the police!

The following are a few examples in my experience.

One Joe Ramharack, aged twenty-seven, came to me one night alleging that he had been beaten by two policemen in a cemetery after he had buried his infant child. I found injuries to his head, ear, eye, mandibles, shoulder blade, elbow, knee and back. At the hearing, I was soundly cross-examined for a total of three hours, and roundly abused and insulted by the crown prosecutor (who defended the policemen). The magistrate dismissed the case. Ramharack appealed. The High Court sent the case back for trial before another magistrate. The same crown counsel repeated his performance, the magistrate apologised to me for the lawyer's behaviour and found the policemen guilty as charged.

In these circumstances, it is understandable that most doctors in Trinidad and Tobago bluntly refuse to examine and treat persons who allege that they have been beaten by the police. Yet, a few doctors do examine and treat such patients and they certainly suffer for their pains.

On 10th June, 1972, Christopher Joseph, aged twenty-five, of Fyzabad, was arrested while feeding his sheep. He was put into a cell at the Fyzabad Police Station, with an Alsatian police dog on a leash, tied to his neck. He was mauled on his arm, elbow and forearm. He was released without charge. When I examined him the next day, he had fifteen dog bites oozing pus. He had been to another doctor who had refused to attend to him, saying that he did not wish to get involved. I reported the matter to the Senior Police Commissioned Officer at the station. No action was taken.

On 25th July, 1973, Abraham Mahmood, aged thirty-two, of Fyzabad, was cuffed, kicked and beaten with gun butts by several policemen on his face, chest, neck, low spine and mandibles. When I examined him, I found thirty-six injuries. He was released by the police without being charged with any offence.

On 24th July, 1973, Peter Chandree, aged twenty-three, of Fyzabad, was beaten with batons and gun butts by policemen, taken to the Oropouche Police Station, made to kneel down and was kicked over, then put into a car, his trousers fly opened and a live crab (crustacean, not pediculous) applied to his genitals. He was put in a cell at the San Fernando police station, handcuffed to a bed, a lighted cigarette applied to his tongue, and he was ordered to swallow the cigarette. When I examined him on 27th July, he had eight bumps on the scalp, injuries to temple, ear, back, chest wall, spine area and thighs. He had a burn on the lower lip. He had been released that day without any charges being laid against him.

On 9th September, 1973, a man came to me at my office and told me that his younger brother whose initials are K.M. (this matter is sub-judice), living at Siparia, was kidnapped by some men in plain clothes. He asked me to investigate this. I phoned the superintendent of police in the area several times with negative results. He said he knew nothing about the young man in question. The next day, *my* house was searched by men armed with sub-machine guns and self-loading rifles, ostensibly for arms and ammunition, and I was arrested at gunpoint. I did not know it, but at the police station I was kept a few yards away from K.M. He came to see me on the fifteenth after his release suffering from pneumonia contracted from exposure in the cell.

I am hoping to hear from my Grenadian colleagues about their experiences with mongoose bites.[10]

Pouring more money into the same inefficient structure can never solve the problems of medical care. Inflation and bottlenecks will only be accentuated.

After over twenty years of examination of the ills and difficulties associated with primary and other medical care, such as related above, the Trinidad and Tobago Medical Association produced a paper embodying recommendations for a full, comprehensive prepaid medical plan.

It is clear that the above plan, if efficiently operated, could solve most of the difficulties of primary and secondary medical care, and so assist in their primary objective: the safeguarding and restoration of the health of the citizen.

But there is another development which is necessary if the best results are to be obtained from any plan regarding human beings, and which is, in fact, mandatory, even if the best plan is not to be abused and on the positive side succeed in giving psychological satisfaction to all participants, the giver and the receiver alike. This is to say, the development of a sense of community.

The Community

Rapid transport and migration from village to town has tended to destroy most of the community spirit and community interest that used to be, and has replaced it with a sort of pseudo-centralisation which has destroyed the aura of friendly contact and personal interest which is as important for many human social activities, including efficient primary care.

It would seem imperative at this stage in the development of Trinidad and Tobago, while there is yet enough physical space available, that we should design a comprehensive plan for the establishment of new communities, based on agricultural, fishing and industrial economic resources, in as many parts of the country as possible. In many instances, it would be possible for many small communities to undergo planned coalescence. Urban communities

---

[10] A reference to the 'Mongoose Gang' of Grenada – similar to the 'Tonton Macoute' of Haiti.

would be even easier to establish. In each community, the hospital and health centre, like the schools, recreation halls, National Service office (NOT the Police Station) with their respective staffs, would be an integral part, belonging to, serving and controlled by the community.

It is fascinating to speculate on the psychological and other medical aspects of such a community: education for public health, nutrition, planning of families and so on would take on new dimensions. The tasks would certainly be far simpler, the satisfactions and rewards more immediate and much more intense.

One thing is certain: in the presence of such a community of economy and of interest, the first part of this paper which I offer to you today, this litany of woes, would in 1986 be quite unnecessary.

Health and the Trinidad and Tobago Economy

(Paper, presented to the African Medical Conference held in Nairobi, Kenya in 1983. Reprinted from the Guardian *and* Express)

Modern science and technology at the end of the twentieth century, appear to have determined that most of the clinical activities of the doctor may be performed much more quickly and efficiently by computers and robots. Let us gratefully and gracefully accept these tools – when our countries can afford them and the unemployment which goes with them. Let us utilise the time thus saved by raising our heads and looking around us, with our uniquely human perspective, at those economic and sociological factors which contribute to health and disease in our environment, because the presence of human emotion – and the phenomenon of caring – the presence of intellect and foresight are the attributes which distinguish us quantitatively from the lower animals and qualitatively from the machine.

The developing country which I have chosen is Trinidad and Tobago, and I have done so for two reasons: first, it is the country which I know best and, second, it is a microcosm in which one finds all the complexities of much larger countries concentrated in a small area, so that to the discerning eye the reasons for success or failure can quickly be ascertained – often before completion.

Our two thousand square miles can be sunk without trace in one tenth of Lake Victoria. We number one and a quarter million souls or one person per acre. Rain falls on every square inch of land in the rainy season, averaging a hundred and forty to three hundred centimetres per annum. The soil is tremendously varied and largely fertile. We have mountains, rolling and level plains, and swamps. Food, of one kind or another, will grow on and in all of these for twelve months of the year. Our marine economic zone of two hundred miles gives us an additional forty thousand square miles which abound with hundreds of species of seafood, and the subsoil of both land and sea is impregnated with petroleum and natural gas.

In this paradise of ours, we have developed a per capita income of some US$4,000 which is much higher than any other developing country. We have a quarter of a million households with one hundred and fifty thousand television sets and radios, we read one hundred and fifty thousand newspapers daily, drive in two hundred thousand motor vehicles – half of them private cars. Each year, we smoke twenty-one million kilograms of cigarettes, drink two million litres of beer, plus two and a quarter million gallons of rum – all three locally manufactured – and we import fifty million dollars worth of whisky, gin, vodka, wines and liqueurs from metropolitan countries. Forty-six per cent of all admissions to hospital are related to alcohol. We are filthily and drunkenly rich.

So much for our God-given wealth and our general usage thereof. How does our health fare? At the start of life, our neo-natal deaths are fifteen per thousand live births – a reflection of our unemployment, underemployment and inadequate housing. The unemployment figure varies with the source of the statistics from fifteen to twenty-five percent of the work force, and these figures are matched by those for underemployment

The incidence of disease related to public health is, according to notifications, one thousand five hundred per annum. From my observations, and those of my colleagues, the figures for gastro-enteritis and hookworm alone would be closer to ten thousand per annum. We have about one hundred thousand cesspits and innumerable open defecating grounds in our country – another index of our filthy richness.

How did our oil wealth contribute to our health? For those of you who need to be reminded, perhaps I ought to give a very brief review of the events associated with the oil boom.

In 1973, the Organisation of Oil Producing Countries, OPEC for short, raised the price of a barrel of crude oil from US$2 to US$17, and later to $34. It occasionally sold at $40. We in Trinidad benefited from this, although we were not a member of OPEC, being as much an importer[11] as an exporter of crude. We used the windfall money to embark on a very extensive programme of public works, a six lane highway, mini-skyscrapers for government offices, a $240 million racing complex and gambling centre to which the highways gave conspicuous access. The huge surpluses from the sale of crude oil were used to purchase a wide variety of consumer goods, food imports alone approach the billion dollar mark – nearly a thousand dollars for each man, woman and child. Little effort was made to boost local food production, and easy money from industry depleted much of the food producing workforce. The surplus petrodollars were used to subsidise imported foods, local gasoline, increased pensions, and to institute a glorified 'dole' system called 'special works' – the speciality being about two hours' work at drain cleaning per day for $40 to $60 with thousands on the payroll and paid, but many physically unaccounted for.

This tremendous injection of dollars into the economy – so much money chasing so few locally produced consumer goods and phantom services – produced the classical inflationary spiral. Prices quintupled for almost everything, and naturally the lower income groups suffered for food, clothing, housing and medical care.

Venereal Disease

The Annual Statistical Digest, from which I obtained most of the figures used in this paper, states that in 1973, free, government clinics diagnosed 1,290 cases of syphilis, 10,451 cases of gonorrhoea, and 4,198 cases of other venereal diseases. In 1978 (after the oil boom started), they diagnosed 1,017 syphilis, 3,028 gonorrhoea, and 4,332 other venereal diseases. The decrease corresponds inversely with a massive increase in private practice, according to the records of my colleagues and myself, because the participants were more affluent they could now afford private treatment. Incidentally, they also paid more to contact and contract the diseases: I am told (strictly hearsay evidence!) that the price before the oil boom varied between $10 and $50; post OPEC it was $50 to $200. These figures are not from the

---

[11] Crude oil imported from Venezuela, Africa and the Far East is refined in Trinidad, and the end products exported to the metropolis.

statistical digest, yet, in that publication the printer's devil has not been idle. One of the blemishes on the noble shrine of Venus is listed as *Nymphogranuloma venerum*!

Motor Accidents

In 1973, there were one hundred and ten thousand motor vehicles on our roads. There were eighteen thousand serious accidents, four thousand causing injuries of which two hundred were fatal. In 1978, there were one hundred and eighty thousand motor vehicles, twenty-six thousand serious accidents, five thousand six hundred and sixty seven injuries, two hundred and thirteen of which were fatal. More affluence, more cars, more alcohol, more injuries, more deaths, a greater workload on medical personnel. Anyone who has worked in a casualty department is aware of the exhausting time and effort required for the diagnosis and treatment and subsequent legal involvement relating to road traffic injuries, to the detriment of equally deserving non-accident cases.

Yet, in our country we have no mass transit systems like electric, or other, trains, hovercraft or hydrofoil to take cars off the road. Traffic jams in Trinidad often exceed two miles, and commuters may take an hour to travel a quarter mile after work, in the city. Quite apart from the frustration and mental imbalance thereby occasioned, the inhalation of exhaust fumes for one to three hours at a time must do incalculable damage to every cell in the human body.

The Aftermath

It is now history that oil prices and demand have fallen, and we are in the middle of a worldwide recession. Trinidad's economy and the health of her population are in deep trouble. The $34 billion earned from oil during the boom gave us a foreign reserve of some $12 billion, and this has dwindled to an estimated $2 billion.

The worldwide recession is not the main cause of our problem. Our weakness lies in our dependence for income on exports to the metropolitan countries, at prices determined by them, and on importing food and other consumer goods from them, again at their prices. We imitated metropolitan industries, copied their technology, often purchasing their cast-off obsolescence. We aped their wasteful, if glamorised, urban lifestyles and misapprehension of values.

How could such a sophisticated people like Trinidadians and Tobagonians commit such errors? There are three main reasons. First, we had been inundated with propaganda, emanating largely from the USA, in favour of this way of life and standards of living – not the rural American standards of massive and efficient production of food surpluses, not the logic consistently espoused by the American based World Watch Institute.

Second: we had always been – as a legacy of the colonial pattern – export and import oriented, with commission agents holding economic power and influencing, even controlling, Government policy.

Third: massive projects provided the opportunity for those in charge of Government agencies to receive substantial finders' fees, commissions, kick backs and occasionally naked bribes, so that policy decisions involving the expenditure of millions, even billions, came to depend to a larger extent on the source and size of the 'commissions' than on the probable advantage to the nation.

Questionable payments have been uncovered in connection with the purchase of wide-bodied aircraft, oil drilling concessions and an unfinished, cost-overrun racing complex. In a celebrated case, a former Government Minister, named in Parliament and in the press, who accepted a 3.6 million dollar bribe was allowed to leave the country with most of his booty and go to live in Panama. In addition, he is being paid a pension for his services.

As it happened, we spent most of our windfall on capital intensive industries instead of agricultural farms, food production and processing which would have given many more people meaningful employment, thereby bolstering their health in mind and body. Our manufacturing industries, as a result of the glut overseas, are dismissing their workers by the hundreds, and our major oil refinery, Texaco, has let over a thousand men go and has offered the company for sale. Because of a depleted treasury, our government has reduced the subsidies on gasoline and several foodstuffs, and raised the price of electricity and telephones. Like King Midas, we are faced with starvation because of the golden touch.

The Lesson for Developing Countries

The lessons, which we in developing countries must learn from all of this, are that our mental and physical health rest firmly and unshirkably on the economics of our respective countries, that affluence is never an unqualified guarantee of good health and may indeed aggravate disease, it is certainly no substitute for proper economic planning based not solely on profit but primarily on the health needs of the people. Last, I hope and trust that my esteemed colleagues here present, who have done me the honour of listening so patiently to the problems of my tiny but beloved nation, should remind themselves that no matter how competently, honestly and sincerely we may practice our profession, we doctors and our patients can easily remain merely victims of a poorly planned economy. Unless we take a more active interest in these basic matters, we may find that we have abandoned our less fortunate fellow citizens to the mercies of opportunists, charlatans and crooks, and while we may save the lives of many people, we may yet lose the population.

(This has been an abridged version of the paper.
Certain portions have been omitted for economy of space.)

When Patients Who Need Transfusion Refuse Blood

(When I was Public Relations Officer of the TTMA, there was a report of a member of a religious group who needed transfusion but refused blood. The following was sent to the press by the PRO desk, and it was reproduced in both daily newspapers.)

Doctors who attended the Annual General Meeting of their Association, on Thursday last, at the General Hospital, San Fernando, were deeply concerned, and expressed their profound sympathy for those patients for whom a blood transfusion could be a matter of life or death, but who, for religious reasons, could not accept blood. In Trinidad and Tobago, members of the Jehovah's Witnesses religion form the majority of people with this religious conviction.

The doctors agreed that the wishes of all minorities – however small the percentage – must be respected. But how to save their lives?

It was pointed out at the meeting that 'artificial blood' is being developed in Japan, and ideally this could be procured by the Ministry of Health for use in such cases. In the meantime, however, especially considering that for one reason or another it is often impossible for patients to get even common medicines at government institutions, and even in-patients have to send out to get the drugs prescribed by the hospital doctor, it would be advisable for religious groups who require 'artificial blood' to keep a small stock available for their members who might need it.

The Ministry, however, should take note that 'artificial blood' is useful in many instances other than refusal to take natural blood. Among these are the following.

Unavailability of compatible blood
Delayed arrival of blood
'Bloodless' surgery – to avoid risk of hepatitis
Carbon monoxide poisoning
To correct lack of oxygen in the brain
To improve coronary circulation in heart muscles
For severe auto-immune haemolytic anaemias
As an oxygen-carrying plasma expander in various kinds of
impaired blood flow.

So that it would be well worthwhile their taking in a stock of this new substance. The trade name is 'FLUOSOL DA', and it is a 20% solution of an emulsified mixture of perfluorodecalin and perfluorotripropylolamine.

(The technical information above is based on a report to the Editor in the October 1982 issue of Medicine Digest, to which journal the PROdesk of the TTMA wishes to express thanks.)

Medical Examination
For Driver's Permit

Persons applying for a permit to drive certain classes of motor vehicles are required to obtain from a doctor, a medical examination reported on the form of medical certificate labelled, 'Licensing-3', which is supplied to them by the Licensing Authority. The motivation behind this requirement is good, and it deserves the support of all citizens of an enlightened country.

Yet, the 'Licensing-3' form had not been designed for the purpose for which it is being used, and for whatever purpose, it falls far short of what it could become if expertly drafted: (1) It is explanatorily subheaded: 'In the case of suspected medical unfitness, it is important that the Licensing Authority be satisfied on the following points before the grant of a driving permit.' It is clear that this form was drafted for the purpose stated above, and, indeed, I have been filling out a similar form for the past twenty-nine years, for drivers with defects of eye or limb obvious to anyone and, therefore, to the clerk at the Licensing Authority.

The only comment to be made regarding this archaic procedure is that when the form was drafted in the dim and distant past – when we were just emerging from the horse and buggy pace and motor car and pedestrian population to match – this form could have served the purpose of appearing to safeguard the driver, his passengers and the person on foot. The fact is, that it only appeared to do so, as I trust will emerge unequivocally from the rest of this contribution.

(2) In paragraph four of the form, under EYESIGHT, we find, (a) Is there a defect of vision? and (b) If a defect of vision is revealed on examination, give acuity of vision by Shellen's (sic) test. [The misspelling of Dr Snellen's name has persisted in hundreds of reprints of this form!] (c) Do you consider that the subject should wear glasses?

Now, a defect of vision – if not obvious to the layman – is detected by the examining doctor, using Snellen's test in the first instance. Many of my colleagues, and myself, have tested applicants who have been driving for many years, and have been given a form only because, under the new regulations, they need it for a goods or other heavy vehicle, and we find that some of these persons can read only the first two rows of letters, (i.e. 6/36 on Snellen's chart), and have driven for years without glasses, which they desperately need in order to drive safely. That person may appear to, and may actually believe that they have perfect eyesight, and their deficiency is detected only after the Snellen's reading test. Most of these applicants are very grateful to their doctor, who has insisted that they get refracted by an optician, and are then passed for driving with glasses. It is clear, therefore, that *all* applicants should be Snellen tested, and that the procedure should not be left to individual discretion.

(3) Field of vision: there are people who have excellent distant vision, and will read down to the last line on Snellen's chart, but cannot see on the sides. Their field of vision is restricted to what is called 'tunnel vision'. The commonest cause of this is glaucoma, and tunnel vision should disqualify a person from driving

(4) Colour vision: this should be tested in view of the present day prevalence of traffic lights.

All the above points were made in a memorandum submitted to the Licensing Authority by the Trinidad and Tobago Medical Association several months ago, and I am personally very disappointed that action has not been taken in this regard.

The Medical Association has, among its members, doctors with a tremendous range of experience. There are few questions, with medical implications under consideration by Government agencies, which cannot be effectively analysed and efficiently commented on by the Association – and I trust that this body will be consulted on all such matters in future, and so avoid public hardship and waste of public funds because the planners did not have the experience in the broad fields of human activity which is really the strongest asset of the Medical Association.

(Note: This is an abridged version of the letter published in the Trinidad Guardian *on 16th May, 1979.*

172

Up to today, 30th April, 1995, the same old obsolete form is still being presented to me by potential drivers!)[12]

---

[12] 'He' is used throughout the form despite the present day prevalence of female drivers!

What Constitutes Incapacity to Do One's Work?

(Paper presented at the Sick Leave seminar on 19th March, 1978)

It has been said, somewhat cynically, of the professional, whether lawyer, engineer, economist, doctor or a devotee of the most ancient profession, that his or her function is so to complicate terminology or technique that in the end the enchanted layman has no alternative but to throw himself blindly and supplicatingly on the practitioner's tender mercies.

For this reason, Mr President, ladies and gentlemen, please be reassured that the purpose of this paper is simply to analyse, not to mesmerise – to clarify, not to confuse.

Firstly, let us consider the basic premise regarding 'capacity for work' or 'ability to work', and enunciate a fundamental principle which I believe would be acceptable to all present here this morning. There are three obvious interdependent factors or forces involved:

(1)   The nature of the work
(2)   The nature of the illness
(3)   The nature of the person – the 'Persona'

The doctor must carefully consider the interplay of these forces, any one of which can, in special circumstances, prove to be the dominant factor. Yet, having made a decision, there are still other factors to be considered, before the medical expert further decides that the person should be permitted to perform his duties.

Let me illustrate, by examples, the workings of this 'infernal' triangle.

The Chief Personnel Officer (who is also a director of the company) has an acute virus infection with blocked up sinuses, pain all over the body and a high fever. He visits his doctor, takes his medicines to ease his symptoms, but refuses to stay off work, only to find on his desk a sick leave certificate from his secretary who had been to the same doctor with the same illness! The obverse phenomena, namely the will to fight, and the retreat into illness, have survival value for different types of individual, and some persons carry in the forefront of their minds the adage, attributed to Napoleon Bonaparte, 'He who fights and runs away/Will live to fight another day/But he who is in battle slain/Will never live to fight again.'

A mild coronary insufficiency would not demobilise a construction engineer, but might incapacitate his labourer for several weeks. Here, the nature of the work is the deciding factor for the identical illness. A business executive whose animal fat and cigarette intake, and emotional output, warrants it, may be strongly cautioned that he had better take his sick leave or risk a massive myocardial infarct. In this instance, the persona is the dominant factor, while the natures of the work and of the illness remain approximately identical with those relating to the engineer. A massive infarct will immobilise all categories of persona and work.

You can multiply these examples endlessly from your own experiences. I am sure that the tremendous resources of courage among you in the audience – if you did not have courage you would hardly be here this Sunday morning after your exhausting Saturday night out! – must determine that you seldom take any sick leave at all, or take it only if you have some seriously incapacitating illness. By the same token, you must know dozens of cases in your own businesses who take all the sick leave to which they are entitled and ask for more.

How then, does the doctor decide on individual cases in this complex triangle of forces?

There are clear cut instances which pose no problem at all: the patient comes up and says: "Doctor, I am not really sick but I want a few days off," or "Boss, how much for a sick leave certificate?", or "I want to repair my house and I must have four days sick leave." The doctor who grants these requests should not be permitted to practise.

One man came to me and told me, "Doctor, I have been your patient for twenty years and my entire family comes to you. I want to ask you a little favour, and I don't mind giving you something for your trouble. My only daughter is graduating in England this week, and I want to attend the graduation, but the only way I can get time off is to give the company a sick leave certificate." I explained that this would be wrong, and that he ought to put his case to the company officials and try in that way to get leave. He replied that perhaps he could do that, but he would not be paid during his absence. I again explained that it would not be right for me to accede to his request, which he again repeated with a few embellishments. Thereupon, he grew serious, and took on a look of disconsolate aggrievement. I tried to make him understand that I could lose my medical practice if I issued a false certificate, but his stand was that, despite his and his family's loyalty to me over two decades, I had refused to help him out. He told me, point blank, that he could easily have got it from Dr X, but only came to me because I was his regular doctor, and he preferred to give me the money rather than give it to another doctor. Now that I had treated him so badly, he would go to X, and neither he nor his family would come to me again. I am sure that my ethics have cost me hundreds, in notes and in votes.

But there are doubtful cases: symptoms without signs – the severe headache, pain in the neck, tightness in the chest, cramps in the abdomen (any of the four quadrants) a history of diarrhoea, with frequent visits to the doctor's toilet in demonstration or remonstration for having to wait his turn. A doctor may spend an hour examining one patient, while those with obvious signs as well as symptoms may be moaning, coughing and groaning in the waiting room. After having written up the patient for various tests, the doctor is still not sure whether he is dealing with some organic disease, hysteria or malingering. His intuitive guess is almost always correct, but he can refuse to give sick leave and to treat on the basis of his intuition, and risk having many sleepless nights by wondering if he had missed a cardiac infarct, an incipient cerebral haemorrhage, an early appendicitis or an ectopic pregnancy. There is, of course, the occasional nightmare in which the doc is in the dock on a malpractice or criminal negligence suit. As Hamlet said, 'To sleep, perchance to dream/Aye there's the rub.'

In view of all this, I have no qualms whatsoever if one of my patients, with a sore throat or gonorrhoea, having taken my medicines and my sick leave certificate, is seen by his boss watching cricket at the Oval. Better that he and I should relax, watch the Australians' balls being knocked about and give the West Indians a hearty clap for their efforts.

A person who does not want to work will get sick leave by hook or by crook: in 1950, as a young and very energetic casualty officer at the Colonial Hospital, San Fernando (yes, we were energetic though colonial), I removed a cyst one morning from the face of a young man at his request, and then, again at his request, gave him a certificate of inability to attend court. I later learned that he had deliberately chosen that morning for the operation, in order to delay affiliation procedures at the court. He had no qualms about keeping the lady waiting, but had I known beforehand, I would certainly have spared the scalpel and helped the child.

Then, there are very deserving cases, but unfortunately not deserving of a *medical* certificate. A consideration of these instances leads naturally into the wider fields of leave from work generally of which sick leave is only one ingredient, and into the realms of the philosophy of employer-worker relationship, into which the doctor is, so often unnecessarily, invited to intrude.

A parent brings his very ill child to the doctor and later requests a sick leave certificate for himself so that he will be paid for his days away from work while he looks after the infant. This parent obviously ought to get compassionate leave with pay, but only a very few employers take this view.

A worker's close relative has died. At present, only a few employers give compassionate or bereavement leave for the wake, the interment and the post funeral rituals. Other employers will, with full knowledge of the events and with sympathetic understanding, accept a sick leave certificate and pay the worker fully for his absent days.

A certain employer tells me that he once received a medical certificate with the diagnosis 'marriage disability' for fourteen days. The man had been on his honeymoon. Perhaps, without benefit of doctor the employer might have been inclined to give this 'patient' compassionate leave. Remember the praying (preying) mantis!

Now a few words about words: the semantics of medical certificates.

Example of Form Supplied by One Insurance Agency

I hereby certify that............................ was examined by me and in my opinion was at the time suffering from
....
In my opinion this patient will remain incapable of work for a period of................ days starting from.................................

The wording is bad for the following reasons:

(1) The diagnosis is asked for. This would be a breach of medical professional confidentiality.
(2) 'will remain incapable of work': why the future tense? A certificate may quite correctly be issued a week or a year after the illness and again the person may be quite capable of work, yet sick leave would be justified.

An illness in a person is never in isolation: a mild case of German measles may not prevent a person from working at maximum efficiency, but if he does mingle at the workplace, he can give someone's unborn child a congenital heart disability by infecting them. His mild mumps can give someone an attack of intense testicular pain, resulting in permanent cosmetic disability. A worker's mild attack of chickenpox can give a most senior executive a two week, acute attack of disabling shingles and the permanent pain of post herpetic neuralgia.

Even the dedicated company director, whom we met on the first page, may initiate the loss of many hundreds of manpower hours, by infecting his less involved staff, and may give the odd one a fatal meningitis or encephalitis.

Doctors would do well, therefore, to insist on sick leave being taken by all persons who may be a danger to their colleagues; either through infection, as described above, or if the illness or the medication would be likely to impair their judgement to the extent that, if engaged in potentially dangerous work, for example working on a scaffold, handling dangerous tools or machinery, or even driving a motor vehicle, they may endanger their own lives or those lives around them.

The wording of the certificate ought therefore to be very simple.

This certifies that .... is ill.
I recommend............ days sick leave commencing.................

And so we seem to have come full circle: it appears that employers will, after all, have to throw themselves on the tender mercies of the professional, not I trust blindly and supplicatingly, but with a clearer comprehension of his problem, and a sympathetic understanding of his limitations. I hope that all doctors will prove to be worthy of this trust.

There is an ancillary issue which is widespread and important enough to be included in this paper: the question of maternity leave. The omnipotent doctor is repeatedly requested by his teacher-patient, to postpone or bring forward the expected date of delivery so that the three months' perinatal leave should not coincide with any part of the normal school vacation periods because, as the expectant mother puts it, "I will lose some of my regular vacation benefit if you put the correct expected date of delivery." Such requests are the rule. Exceptions are few, since there are roughly only three months of work between vacation periods. Now, it would take skilled, almost computer-like, planning of conception, to neatly fit normal maternity leave into one of these three months, or, alternatively, the reduction of the gestation period to rabbit-like proportions.

But it is usually the doctor who, rabbit-like, complies with this request. If most doctors were to refuse, the Public Service Association and the Teachers' Union would quickly ensure that some financial adjustment is made for teachers so affected, and the same is true for compassionate leave.

This paper could comfortably end here, but if it did, we would be ignoring the entire context in which the difficulties regarding sick leave have their genesis. We would be technicians, not teachers, as our honorary appellation implies. We would be the objects and puppets of history, not masters of our own destiny as citizens of an independent nation. Let us, therefore, in conclusion, look very briefly at some of the basic contexts of our psycho-sociological development.

Our immediate ancestor in this country, the slave, was exempted from work in his owner's fields only when flat on his back because of illness. I am told that women were often also exempted if placed in a similar position. The indentured labourer was flogged if found outside his master's plantation – unless he could produce a pass, more often than not a pass to go to hospital. It will take more than the passive passing of a few hundred years to eliminate this master-servant psychology, in the absence of a conscious and concerted drive towards true identification of the worker with the proceeds of his work.

It must also be quite clear to you, that nearly all the difficulties associated with the sick leave certificate stem from the existing adversarial relationship which persists between employer and worker, instead of partnership and mutual understanding. Indeed, it was a series of massive 'sick outs' which inspired the current legislation. Still, we have employers who with monotonous persistence throw the burden of decision entirely on the doctor, and regularly attempt to make him the convenient scapegoat for their own shortcomings.

Let them realise that lack of appreciation, motivation and mutual identification is the primary reason why some people can take fourteen days sick leave because they are too ill with bronchitis or rheumatics to dig the government's roads, and then proceed to dig their own fields twice as hard and three times as long with marked improvement to their mental, physical and financial well-being.

In the long run, the true answer to what is a real sick leave problem afflicting our nation, is a greater spread of ownership of the means of production among the rank and file of our citizens, and I throw this out as a subject for research. We already have in some businesses this kind of approach – shares in the company, worker management and so on, and a comparative study would certainly be of interest. I trust that this paper has succeeded in its primary task, namely to stimulate further thought and discussion regarding an important aspect of the utilisation of our resources, indeed, our most important resource, our men and women.

Analysis of Sick Leave Requested by my Patients

(1)   So sick that they cannot work.
(Usually obvious to any layman).   50%
(2)   Have an infectious or contagious disease.
Can work but should not. (Usually obvious,
except where affected organ is hidden).   5%

(3)   Feeling sick enough to stay at home, but with no clinical signs of illness, and with symptoms galore.   7%

(4)   Persons looking and feeling fit, and are clinically healthy, but request sick leave for:

(a) Taking a holiday   5%

(b) Having already taken a holiday without leave   2%

(c) Attending to urgent domestic matters e.g. getting married, taking wife or child to doctor, repairing house, attending funeral, going for driver's permit, attending son's or daughter's graduation abroad, attending or not attending court, attending cricket at the Oval, playing Carnival   10%

(d) Work protest – so called 'sick out'.   ½%

(5)   Persons wanting all the sick leave to which they are entitled, otherwise they would lose it. Usually an end of year epidemic of 'illness'.   20%

99½%

TTMA Considers the Mount Hope Site Unsuitable for a University Complex

The Cabinet of the Government of Trinidad and Tobago, has appointed a task force to consider certain aspects of the proposed building of a teaching hospital and science complex at Mount Hope. Their terms of reference do not include any consideration regarding the suitability of the Mount Hope site for such a project, or the consideration of any alternative site. It is the view of this writer, and of the overwhelming majority of doctors who have considered the question, that Mount Hope presents numerous limitations and disadvantages, and would be one of the worst possible choices for such a complex. It is also the view of the association, that a site in the Ward of Chaguanas would, for the reasons enumerated later in this article, offer such advantages as would make a choice of site in that area irresistible for anyone with the welfare of future generations of our citizens at heart.

The task force has enumerated the following to be included in the complex: a teaching hospital, nursing school, engineering school, agricultural school, facilities for training in ancillary sciences related to the above, laboratories, workshops, dormitories, residences, recreational facilities, fields and other amenities and perquisites necessary for such activities.

It is difficult to understand why the Mount Hope site was considered in the first instance. However, the following alleged advantages have been listed: proximity to the present teaching hospital at Port of Spain, proximity to the proposed maternity hospital at Mount Hope, proximity to the University of the West Indies at St Augustine, proximity to large centres of population for teaching material.

A brief glance at a map of Trinidad, reveals the obvious corollary to the proximities listed above, namely remoteness from the rest of Trinidad to animal populations for veterinary activity, to extensive diversified agriculture, to large scale hydrocarbon and engineering works, and, especially in connection with the teaching hospital, to the very wide ranges of medical and surgical material available from the endeavours listed above.

Again, mere physical proximity is effectively negated by the location of Mount Hope, at the vortex of almost interminable traffic congestion from all four points of the compass.

We have been told that about twenty-five acres are immediately available, and that fifty acres can be added when needed. Expansion beyond this is physically impossible, and it would be lunacy to start such a project, in 1979, on a site so hamstrung by fixed physical boundaries. This fact, and that of the cost at present, and the spirally inflating price of lands in the area (with the naturally dependent costs of accommodation and services), should, at the outset, have been important considerations in rejecting as hopeless, the choice of this mount.

What then would be a more ideal location? Where in Trinidad can we find a site which possesses nearly all the advantages of Mount Hope, none of the disadvantages, and all of the attributes required by such a complex?

A site in the Ward of Chaguanas, embracing possibly Carlsen Field. This site is approximately fifteen miles long, from its eastern tip near the centre of Trinidad to its western shore on the Gulf of Paria. It is about twelve miles wide, from north to south along the Churchill-Roosevelt Highway, which traverses it roughly at the junction of its western and middle thirds. Most of it is flat or gently sloping land, and well drained with a firm foundation. A number of square miles is owned or controlled by the government through Caroni Limited and formerly US leased Carlsen Field.

The centre of the Ward of Chaguanas is about fifteen miles from St Augustine (and Mount Hope), fifteen miles from Point Lisas, and ten miles from the Tabaquite tunnel, once the gateway of our railway through the Central Range, and the penetration of this watershed – a geographical and psychological concept – provided an important connecting link between the remote south east and proximal north-west of the Island.

Due south, are the Montserrat Hills and valleys, containing one of the most fertile soils in the world, and some of its lofty outcrops provide a breathtaking panorama of the Northern and Southern Ranges, and of Point Lisas and the Gulf of Paria. Much of this is government owned Forres Park Estate.

In a complex which aims to satisfy the needs of such a wide range of activities as outlined by the task force – and which indeed are vitally important for the future development of Trinidad and Tobago and the rest of the Caribbean – one must envisage a university town with dimensions of about two square miles or about one thousand two hundred acres, not a measly fifty acres. The present writer was a student between 1936 and 1939 at the Imperial College of Tropical Agriculture, whose one hundred or so acres were beautifully and efficiently laid out and utilised for a school of agriculture alone, alas – British imperialist and colonialist! But, we have all witnessed with sorrow the hideous desecration of this acreage with a stifling aggregation of masonry – fitting monuments to the short-sightedness of our planners, and the apathy of the new Caribbean man. This must not happen again.

One thousand two hundred acres in the Ward of Chaguanas would offer, quite literally, newer and broader vistas for architectural and engineering planning. The task force envisages several four-storey buildings, at tremendous dollar-per-floor area cost, a necessity in a restricted ground area such as Mount Hope. In the university town of Chaguanas, land area would be no problem and it would be easy to plan lovely, durable efficient colonies of one or two-storey buildings, at relatively low cost garnished with beautiful lawns, parks, recreation areas and agricultural fields.

In spite of this elbow room the location will be roughly only half an hour from Port of Spain and San Fernando by existing highway, and will be practically on the doorstep of the industrial development at Point Lisas. The availability of an airfield nearby (built during the second world war by the Americans) is another advantage.

In striking contrast with Mount Hope, there will be sufficient land cheaply available for the establishment of all the supportive and service industries necessary for the complex, and it would be quite unnecessary to depend on the expensive facilities already existing in a highly urbanised and overcrowded society.

One can foresee a university community, free from the harassment of pedestrian and traffic congestion, supported by agricultural production, experimental factories, shops, residences, and a complete range of recreational facilities at reasonable cost to students and the community, and in a large measure insulated from the jungle of inflation and community chaos surrounding Mount Hope.

Finally, with a nucleus of five hundred acres on the plains of Chaguanas, and a remaining five hundred acres earmarked for expansion, what would be more natural than an invitation to the proposed National Institute for Higher Education and National Institute for Sport, to make the university town their home ?

*(Reprinted from the Caribbean Medical Journal
Volume 40, Nos 1 &2, 1979)*

The Doctor in Politics

(This is an abridged version, published as part of the author's series of political 'Reflections' in the Trinidad Guardian *of 17th and 18th December 1989, of a paper read to the Southern Branch of the Trinidad and Tobago Medical Association at the Trinidad-Tesoro Medical Centre at Santa Flora on 11th June, 1981)*

The doctor in politics is the medical practitioner who is consciously, and more or less actively, engaged in attempting to move the Government from power, or in keeping them there.

The 'Independent Senator' may be regarded as an exception. This limitation in definition is necessary because everyone is in politics whether or not he is aware of it, and whether or not he likes it. A doctor who secretly supports or opposes the government, is taking a political stance, a doctor who says that he cares nothing about politics, is also taking a political stance – apathy being the meat of tyrants. Yet, neither of these can be regarded as being 'in' politics. 'In' must be reserved for the doctor who offers himself for service in the political field.

Doctors have been in politics all over the world, and at all periods of history, with varying ideologies, in government and in opposition, successful and unsuccessful. We have had several good examples in Trinidad: Dr A.A. McShine (Dr Halsey McShine's father), an outstanding nominated member of the Colonial Legislative Council; Dr Tito P. Achong was mayor of Port of Spain; Dr Vilain was mayor of San Fernando; Drs Pat Solomon, Winston Mahabir and Max Awon as members of the Cabinet; Drs Ada Date, Romesh Mootoo, Alexander Sinanan, Michael Beaubrun, Emmanuel Hosein and Wahid Ali as Senators; Drs Forrester, Horace Charles and Winston Williams as elected members of the Lower House of Parliament; and some others, like Drs Aldwyn Francis, Elton Richardson, James Dube, Ivan

Perot and Martin Sampath who have fought and also ran – some perhaps to fight another day!

David Pitt[13], who unsuccessfully sought election in Trinidad, migrated to England and as Lord Pitt – member of the British House of Lords – succeeded the Prince of Wales as President of the British Medical Association.

At present there are at least six practising doctor/politicians: W. Ali, Michael Beaubrun, Romesh Mootoo, Winston Williams, Emmanuel Hosein and myself. An analysis reveals that, out of every hundred doctors, one is or has been active in politics, and this is about the national average for all educated adult citizens.

Now, doctors are a specially qualified group: of all professionals they undoubtedly have the most intimate contact with the ills of human beings – not only 'medical' ills – and are strategically placed to understand the influence of social, economic and political factors on these maladies and on their alleviation.

In addition, they are practical men and women who are called upon (and usually readily respond) to make vital decisions, and act upon them dozens of times every day. And, very importantly, their occupation makes them – potentially and often actually – economically independent.

Why then, do not many more doctors enter active politics when their country today is languishing, and our national resources are being squandered, largely because of the absence of this type of person in politics?

Here are some of the answers which have been given to me.

(1) Medicine and politics do not mix.
(2) A doctor should not enter politics because
     (a) It will interfere with his practice as he will not have the time.
     (b) People do not like to go to a doctor who is engaged in politics.
(3) I am happy as I am. Why should I take on headaches?
(4) I like the government as it is.

---

[13] Lord Pitt died in England, on 17th December, 1994.

(5) If I went into politics it would be to change the government
      but I am afraid of harassment by the police and of harassment
      of my family by supporters of the other side.

All the above are valid, up to a point, but if you analyse the
personalities of the doctors who have gone into active politics, you
will find that their histories reveal an interest in public and political
matters before they became doctors, and in medical politics as soon as
they began doctoring, while those who give the answers enumerated
above, have, in general, retreated into medicine as into an apparently
safe fortress inoculated against – if not actually isolated from – the
heat and dust of a nation in turmoil: enclave citizens, so to speak.

I trust that by making the above statements I have not converted all
my doctor friends into mere colleagues by this time.

Let us examine some of the problems which appear to face the
doctor in politics: I speak largely from my own experience, and I
hope that other doctors in politics will be able to give us the benefit of
their own.

Competition for the Doctor's Time

At first glance, this appears to be a formidable obstacle. Let us
remind ourselves of the thousands of minutes interspersedly spent
doing nothing. It takes only a little organisation to eliminate these
minutes, and give oneself an extra hour and a half each day. Such
organisation involves the training of staff, patients and the doctor
himself. Do you know that there is an average of three minutes
between patients in a doctor's surgery, and this can be reduced to
thirty seconds by an alert receptionist?

So much for physical time, but there is another more intriguing
process which is readily called into operation with a little practice.
That eminent scientist and novelist H.G. Wells, author of *The Time
Machine*, wrote a less well known story which describes how his
hero, by taking a certain drug, was able to live through the interstices
of time so that for him the world around moved in slow motion. But
the human brain can engage in multiple pursuits at the same time
without the use of drugs and I have found that it was easy to consider
aspects of a political topic one evening, and while it gestated in my

mind subconsciously, during my medical practice, I could, immediately after lunch set down a complete resumé, with recommendations in note form!

If I had to speak on a political platform at say seven in the evening, additions and punchlines would suggest themselves during my talks with my afternoon patients.

The human brain is a wonderful super-computer. All, you have to do is to let it work for you – at the sub-conscious level. At the conscious level, clinical cases are often the catalyst for a political trend of thought: the immunisation of a child suggests a more efficient registration campaign; scabies and nephritis – community water supply and school hygiene. Billions of brain cells work in the nation's interest, while routine medical tasks are performed by just a few million, almost by conditioned reflex, sensitised by years of practical experience, to earn the doctor his daily bread.

So much for the mind; what about the body? This is truly the weaker link, however willing the spirit may be. A reliable secretary, motor car and driver, are great assets, but physical weaklings can forget about being a doctor in active politics. It is much easier for the bodies of politicians in power, who can rest their bodies while the full force of television can do much of their work for them, but for those who strive to capture the citadel, it is a task of Churchillian dimensions: literally blood, sweat and toil, on the beaches, in the fields, on the streets, and often in the homes – tears.

Conflict of Interest

This is a real and moral factor. In 1958, after Dr Williams' very unstatesmanlike pronouncement in Woodford Square, about the 'recalcitrant minority', set the seal on Africans versus Indians at all future elections, it was predicted that as a PNM candidate I would lose all my Indian patients!

Some mischievous people on the Opposition DLP platform announced that Dr Williams had instructed all Indian PNM doctors to give a sterilising injection to all Indian women so as to limit the Indian population! As a result, I started getting numerous requests from ladies of all races for this particular injection! I did lose many of my

Indian clientele, but they all came back when the election fever and its debilitating aftermath were forgotten.

My impression is that the politics of a doctor do not permanently affect his practice. People will come to you if they think that you are a good doctor, but will vote as they wish (usually for the party 'of their own race') when elections come around. It would be presumptuous for any doctor to hope that because of his popularity as a medico, his patients would vote for him.

Like the rest of the population, the medical fraternity has its full share of opportunists and cowards, but in politics we have to accept people as they are, not as we would like them to be. In practising the art of the possible, we must find (to paraphrase the immortal bard) tongues in trees, books in the running brooks, sermons even in 'millstones' (as Dr Williams once categorised some of his Ministers): *As You Like It*.

My Medical Colleagues

When I was among eleven persons arrested and jailed for marching, I posed this question to some of my medical colleagues: "If I were convicted and sent to jail, would you protest?" One close friend among them replied unhesitatingly, "Martin, boy, I am sorry to say that your 'friends' would do nothing to help you. Some of them would be only too happy to see you out of circulation so that they could grab your patients!"

When the Medical Association, as a body, criticised the Speaker of the House of Representatives for allowing the confidential medical records of an airline pilot to be read in open Parliament, and broadcast live over radio and television, the Speaker threatened to jail us if we had the temerity to repeat our objections. We kept our respective and respectable tails between our legs, despite my own individual recommendation. It is my view that we let down the profession and the country on that occasion very badly: we should have voiced our objection again, and gone to jail *en masse* in support of our stand. But, I suppose that most doctors did not care to relinquish their practices to their more 'discreet' colleagues in our noble profession.

It is clear that doctors individually, and as a group, must always attempt to analyse the motives of politicians, even if they themselves are not actively engaged in politics. No one is politically neutral. Neutrality is but a mirage and often a cloak for cowards. (Now I know that I have lost all my doctor friends).

In 1981, we old stagers observed with pleasure the persistent efforts of our junior colleagues to improve conditions of work. They deserved our support, despite the occasional feeling of *déjà vu*. Some of us in my generation, in testing our own courage almost to its limits, and failing, I like to imagine because in the slow grinding of the wheels of the Gods, the time for success had not arrived, might be permitted to survive long enough to see the heroic efforts of these young men and women crowned with victory.

I am sure that we all look forward to seeing them succeed as doctors, as doctors in medical politics, and a few of them as doctors in active national politics.

Women's Travails
and Triumphs

Puberty, Pregnancy and Menopause

The timing of the onset and final cessation of menstruation varies widely. I have not detected any correlation with race or state of nutrition, perhaps because in this country there are no cases of gross malnutrition such as one has observed in concentration camps.

There is some indication that girls follow the patterns of their mothers. This is relatively easy to detect, since young girls usually come to the doctor accompanied by the female parent, and even if the father were present, it is very unlikely that he would know about his mother's or sisters' history. Yet it would be a worthwhile investigation to discover the genetic antecedents of the onset and cessation of these episodes.

Morning sickness definitely follows the mother's pattern. I have observed that whereas some ladies vomit a great deal for pregnancies which turn out to be male, and hardly at all for female foetuses, the opposite is also true. The belief that there is a hormonal input in the phenomenon of hyperemesis gravidarum thus appears to have support, but it is unclear why the foetus' sex has the opposite effect on different women.

Some of my patients who started bleeding at the age of nine, have gone on to have their menopause at fifty-five, while those who started at thirteen or fourteen, are finally free of encumbrances in their early forties.

One lady of fifty-two had had no menses for three months. We both thought it was menopause, but a routine examination including a urine pregnancy test revealed an unexpected occasion for celebration. She had been married for thirty years to the same husband and had never been pregnant. She had a completely uneventful gestation and was delivered by Caesarean at the appropriate time.

That was my oldest pregnant patient: my youngest was aged eleven.

Contraception and Abortion

I get requests for performing abortions, on average, once per fortnight. Ninety-five percent of these are from married mothers with 'too many children already'. One of these had fourteen alive out of eighteen pregnancies. These days (1990s), most requests come from ladies with three to five children. My advice to all, married and unmarried, is to have the baby and to tie the tubes soon afterwards. Most of them go elsewhere to have the abortion induced, and, significantly, nearly all of them come back to me either for a related condition or something completely unrelated. The point is that I have not lost a single patient by refusing to do an abortion. Without prompting, they usually tell me who did the job for them, but these doctors need not be apprehensive: I believe that the request for abortion arises out of economic stress in married women and out of shame in unmarried ones. Society is savage in this respect and the ostracism meted out to these unfortunate girls, and the use of the word 'illegitimate' on birth certificates, is a barbarous manifestation of human cruelty.

Without exception, all those mothers and grandparents who have taken my advice and continued with their pregnancies, have come back to me with gratitude for my guidance. The happiness which these babies have brought to the families in which they were born is remarkable. Those with multiple progeny tell me, "Doctor, this is the best and most loving child of all."

Domestic Violence

(The following is an abridged version of my contribution in the Senate on the Domestic Violence Bill of March 1991, reproduced in the Sunday Guardian *)*

In my practice, I see approximately one case per week of domestic violence. One case per week is about fifty cases per year, so that I could say that I have seen about two thousand cases of domestic violence in my own short lifetime.

The cases I am going to present today are recent cases. I am presenting these cases because I had the opportunity of asking these victims, "How is it that this happened?" One of them was a girl whom I had delivered, so I knew her for her whole lifetime. She was now twenty-five, married for five years, with two children. She was slapped heavily over the eyes, and had a contused retina. Her reading was three lines less than with the unaffected eye.[14]

"Why did he lash you?"

"We had an argument about something, and I answered him back."

Most of the cases of domestic violence that I have seen are cases where the wife is intellectually superior to the husband, so that she wins nearly every argument, and the husband angrily resorts to force. It is almost like what happens in the wider world: violence and war being an extension of what cannot be done by diplomacy! [Addendum on 18th September 1994: Witness Presidents Clinton, Carter and others on Haiti!]

A twenty-six year old woman came to me on February 21st. Her face was swollen all over: her husband had cuffed her.

"With one hand or both?"

"With both hands like a punching bag."

They had four children, the eldest was five, the youngest was one. This was about the twentieth time that she had been attacked, cuffed and kicked. She had a swollen scalp and face, scratches and marks on the neck, her voice was hoarse: she had been throttled.

These women come to me in tears: here is someone who they love and he beats them – the mental violence is greater even than the severe physical violence. So it is a terrible thing, this wife beating.

"Why did he beat you?"

"Well, he accused me of having a relationship with the neighbour."

"What did he actually say?"

---

14 In the Snellens's reading chart set at six metres, each line has letters smaller than in the line above. This patient's damaged eye could read only the first four lines, while her undamaged eye could read seven lines.

"He said that I was brushing with the neighbour."

You see, the use of words is very important. The word she used suggested an affectionate relationship, and the husband thought he was losing her affection to someone else.

Some people suspect infidelity, but have no proof, then some little thing happens in the house, like dropping a tea cup or making a sharp remark, and the husband resorts to violence, to take revenge for the suspected infidelity.

A woman of twenty was brought to me by her parents. Her injuries had been inflicted by the flat surface of a cutlass – a 'planass', (from the Spanish 'plano' – flat and 'assier' – to assault).

In the olden days, when a cocoa planting contractor came home from the fields, he expected certain things, and if the house was untidy or the children unkempt or food not on the table, if he was in a foul mood, he planassed his wife. If he found her in bed with another man, he gave her the cutting edge.

People ask me, "Why do they not defend themselves when they are getting the flat side of the blade?"

Obviously, if the man is wielding a cutlass, he has her at his mercy. He is at that instant a man possessed with an exquisite sense of power. He can be cruel, if he wishes, and merciful at the same time, because with a small inclination of his mind and the blade, he could do irreparable damage to his victim.

There are several reasons why men beat their female companions. One is frustration at work: a violent man comes home, and argues with his partner about any little thing, and beats her as the whipping girl for his boss. She may be submissive, so, when the man is away, his children become the whipping boys and girls for their father.

There is a thread running through all this: each victim tells me about the husband and the husband's family. "Her man," they say, "beat her when he was drunk, *just like his father used to beat his mother.*" So there is an aetiological factor in domestic violence. The reason for domestic violence is that couples – especially the female partner – do not know, before they get together, what role they are expected to play in the partnership. Many women tell me: "Doctor, if I only knew that he was like that, I would never have married him."

So while the Domestic Violence Bill is important, it is equally important that investigation of the partner's family and of his or her own habits and temperament should be pursued before taking the plunge.

Is Nuclear Energy Worthwhile?

(Reprinted from the Sunday Guardian *25th May, 1986)*

When the world first embarked on the production of electricity through steam generated by the heat of nuclear fission, in the mid-1950s, it was envisaged that nuclear or atomic energy would provide, for all mankind, a clean, safe source of power, for rich and poor alike. It was said in some quarters that the only unsound aspect of the new technology was that there would be little money to be made from it because the electricity thus produced would be 'too cheap to be metered'.

The recent disaster at Chernobyl, in the Soviet Union, which is perhaps only the greatest of more than a dozen smaller ones distributed over the nuclear world, has demonstrated with chilling clarity that nuclear energy is far from safe.

And, now that more than four hundred nuclear plants have been in operation for several years, economists have revealed that electricity from this source is the most expensive ever produced.

It is important that we, in this little country, should be aware of the important factors associated with the use of nuclear energy before pressures are brought to bear upon us to introduce this technology into our as yet non-nuclear polluted environment.

The dangers of nuclear energy begin at the source: when uranium is mined, the workers are exposed to radiation. This would not concern us here, as we have no uranium deposits. We would probably be encouraged to buy enriched uranium, in the form of ceramic pellets sealed in metallic fuel rods, by high powered salesmen from the United States, Canada or South Africa, working in league with nuclear reactor salesmen from Canada or West Germany.

Even if we had extremely corrupt government officials, it is unlikely that these salesmen would succeed, because of the abundance of cheap natural gas available to us – but we could be very susceptible in about thirty years' time when our supply of cheap methane will be exhausted. But countries like Jamaica, must, at this time, be on guard against such blandishments.

The danger begins here: misplacement-pilferage of the radioactive material.

The second danger is the leakage of water, used to cool the core of the reactor. This is known in the trade as LOCA (loss of coolant accident), and has actually occurred in some reactors. The core melts and destroys the containment vessel, and the resulting radioactivity converts the surrounding countryside into a death trap.

The third danger is the disposal of the inevitable radioactive waste. This is already a tremendous and virtually unsolveable problem all over the nuclear world. This consideration alone should deter us from any thought of introducing a nuclear energy reactor here.

Sometimes I wonder how many of the unexplained fish kills we have had, with millions of carcasses afloat and washed up on our beaches, are the result of leaks in the canisters of radioactive waste, known to have been dumped into the sea from nuclear plants.

A nuclear plant is generally expected to have a life of thirty years or less, but even after five years the build-up of radioactivity poses a threat to workers in the plant. There are now more than fifteen plants in the world awaiting decommissioning: some of these are only fourteen years old, yet because of the hazard of radioactive build-up, they are considered to be too dangerous to continue in operation.

The cost of decommissioning a nuclear plant varies from $200 million to $1 billion for a one thousand megawatt reactor. The reason for the high cost is that unlike the demolishing of any ordinary factory, it cannot be just knocked down and transported away as rubble, but it must be cut up by remote control and by workmen who are specially protected.

The fragments must then be transported in specially insulated containers to the burial ground, and when buried must be insulated against radiation escape beneath thousands of tons of concrete and other material. The site will then be out of bounds for thousands of years.

It is clear that, after sober reflection on all the factors mentioned above (perforce so very briefly), no nation should even consider the use of nuclear energy for the generation of electricity. Why then do they?

It is a difficult question to answer. Yet, when one considers that a by-product of the fission of Uranium 235 is Plutonium 239 – a major ingredient of an atomic bomb, it seems that the propensity for nuclear bomb supremacy between the super powers, and the acquisition of nuclear bombs by smaller nations, must be a factor in determining that nuclear fission as a source of energy continues to be pursued.

It is not only a sobering, but a terribly frightening thought to reflect that using an implosion technique, the critical mass for a Plutonium 239 bomb is only four pounds. Just think what a malicious thief or a terrorist could do if he gained access to this 'waste' from a nuclear plant!

When one considers that Providence has already given to mankind – apart from the enormous deposits of fossil fuel (coal, oil and natural gas) which we exploit with extravagant, polluting abandon – a ready made nuclear reactor, our sun, at a safe distance from earth, suitably insulated by a protective shield of two hundred miles of air, we humans must indeed be crazy to enter the dangerous field of nuclear energy, instead of exploiting and developing to its fullest capacity the use of solar energy, which is clean, safe and 'too cheap to be metered'.

TTMA Inaugural and Honours Dinner at Soong's Great Wall Restaurant on 15th January, 1989

Vote of thanks by Dr Martin Sampath
(Reprinted from CMJ *Vol 50, Nos 1 & 2, 1989)*

Your Excellency, Minister of Health, Mayor of San Fernando, Outgoing and Incoming Presidents of the Trinidad and Tobago Medical Association, and charming spouses at the high table and elsewhere.

It is a great pleasure for me this evening, to move the vote of thanks on behalf of the Association. The mover of a vote of thanks is like the junior surgeon at an operation. After the major part of the operation is complete, the senior moving quickly to the adjoining theatre says to his assistant: "Doctor, will you close up please". So I am engaged in the closing ceremony! But the incoming President, with his usual thoroughness, has already done part of the job for me by thanking many of our guests and workers, so it is left for me only to insert the few remaining sutures of my own design – and I promise not to keep you in stitches throughout my contribution.

It is customary to start thanking those at the high table and then to work down gently to the plebeians, but, for variety, I shall do it the other way around on this occasion. Your Excellency, do not be misled by the jackets and ties we have donned tonight: we are all very plebeian here. Whatever the origins of our ancestors from all the continents of the globe, we are of the earth-earthy, our roots are firmly entrenched in the soil of Trinidad and Tobago. There are no transients here.

I myself have on this neck-tie, only because as I was getting dressed I made as if to put on a shirt-jac, but my better half firmly threatened that if I did not resist that impulse, it would be the Last Temptation of Martin![15]

Let me first of all thank the proprietors of this restaurant for the elegant and efficient services of their hostesses, their mien and their menu: rice and tasty buffalypso from Caroni (1975) Ltd, and shrimp from our own Gulf of Paria. If this fine example of local food is intensively and extensively followed, we should save sufficient foreign exchange for Dr Steve Smith to get sufficient US dollars, British pounds, Deutchmarks and Swiss and French francs to purchase all the drugs he needs.

It is my hope that, situated as you are at the 'Great Wall', that is to say at the foot of this unique Naparima Hill, you can be the nucleus of a consortium of hotel keepers and restaurateurs coming together for the establishment of a first class hotel at the top, so that citizens and tourists may relax and enjoy a beautiful panorama of our country – to the economic benefit, naturally, of this new city of San Fernando.

Most of us, in our youth, have also contributed, if not our blood and tears, but at least our sweat and other secretions and excretions to the Hill, so that with the inevitable recycling by nature's persistent vegetation, we too have achieved a certain immortality in the region!

I thank you, my colleagues, for supporting this function in such strength. I interpret this as a demonstration of solidarity.

I thank the recipients of honour scrolls, not only for accepting, but also for the years of dedicated service to humanity which determined our selection of you.

I thank those who introduced you. I realise that it is difficult to be brief when extolling the virtues of your friends. I understand the frustrations of Dr Ram Mahabir. Perhaps we should all take a more active part in politics, instead of passively remaining the frustrated non-recipients of political decisions. Please permit me to quote from memory, something I said in Nairobi as a representative of this Association, at an International Medical Conference there: "You, as doctors, should take an active part in the politics of your country, otherwise you will be at the mercy of charlatans and crooks, and you may personally save many lives, and yet lose the population."

---

[15] An allusion to the then current movie, *The Last Temptation of Christ*, banned in Trinidad and Tobago.

And now for the occupants of the high table: thank you Mr Minister. You will be blamed for many of the sins of your predecessors, but I know that your back is broad and you can take it.

Thank you Mr Mayor for identifying once more with all the activities in your city.

Your Excellencies: you typify all that is noble in our hearts and minds; you are examples of the heights which can be reached by any citizen in our country, whatever his or her origin or the status of their parents. I thank you for coming.

I thank you one and all.

TTMA Installation and Honours Function at the Hilton Hotel on February 11th, 1984

Laudatory Oration for Dr Charles Roderick Thomson
by Dr Martin Sampath, Past President

To compress five decades of excellence, achievement and service into the five minutes allotted to me, is a formidable task: the result has been a virtual implosion of significant facts and indelible impressions which I now present to Dr Thomson's many friends and colleagues assembled here this evening.

His father was the eminent solicitor Charles Caesar Thomson, and his mother was Pamphelia Thomson. He was born on 12th April, 1928, in Port of Spain, and received his early education at Belmont Boys' Intermediate School and St Mary's College. In 1947, he decided that medicine was to be his future calling and while awaiting admission to medical school, he worked at Barclays Bank DCO in the city. In 1948, he became one of the first, and pioneer, batch of thirty-three medical students of the University of the West Indies, and later transferred to University College, Dublin, of the National University of Ireland, graduating with the MB, Ch.B, BAO, in 1957. For the next two years, he served in six British hospitals, and, in 1959, armed with a wealth of clinical experience, he returned to Trinidad, serving for four months as house officer at the General Hospital, Port of Spain. He then entered private practice while serving as Police Surgeon, Physician to the Wharf Clinic and Casualty Officer at the Port of Spain Hospital. In 1962, he became a medical officer for Texaco, working both at Pointe-a-Pierre and at Forest Reserve, and is now Medical Superintendent of Texaco, Trinidad.

He has been a member of the Council of the Medical Board, from 1977 to the present time, and was Chairman of the Committee which assessed the facilities for the training of interns at our hospitals.

He has been a member of the Council of the Trinidad and Tobago Medical Association, since 1970, Chairman of the Southern Division in 1977, and has held the important posts of Chairman of the Ethics Committee, the Primary Health Care Committee, the Watchdog Committee, and the Editorial Committee of the Caribbean Medical Journal.

He was elected President of the Trinidad and Tobago Medical Association for 1981. Notwithstanding his having reached and served at this pinnacle with distinction, he continues to work for the Association and the wider cause of medicine, with his customary youthful zeal and dedication, and continues to be a live wire in committees and delegations, the latest and current being a proposed twenty-four hour health care service for the community.

He is President of the Rotary Club of San Fernando, and is the devoted father of a young man, aged twenty-eight, and twin daughters, aged twenty-three.

Roderick is a well-rounded person – a complete man – yet the symbols of his status are much more than the achievements listed above: his preparation, and the Association's publication, of a code of ethics for medical practice are a landmark in Trinidad and Tobago medical history. His objective and analytical mind has led him to publish numerous articles on forensic medical topics in the *Caribbean Medical Journal* and in the daily press. It is a measure of the man, and his sense of rightness and responsibility that despite the prestigious position from which he is able to speak and write, he has always consulted with other senior members of the Association's Council on his drafts before submitting the final for publication, even when there was urgent need for the correction of published misrepresentation of medical matters or a quick therapeutic abortion of a media misconception.

One could say, in view of the frequently paediatric statements by ostensibly learned friends in other professions and in the administration, that we have prevented the complete spoiling of the child because we have never spared the 'Rod'.

Roderick Thomson is Vice-President of the South Trinidad Music Association. He has an extensive library of recordings, from rare classics to modern jazz. He is a virtuoso at the organ: an electronic model in his living room performs wonders at his fingertips. He does not indulge in horse racing, cock fighting or gambling – unlike one of our other presidents (of the Medical Association). Roderick is a man with music in his soul, and dwelling in the concourse of sweet sounds, he is completely unfit for treason, stratagems and spoils.

He is an exemplar of a now rare gentility, of a nobility which recognises its obligations, and is often the calm centre of many a verbal committee storm, and in all this he is perfectly complemented by his charming, adorable and exuberant wife, Dr Roma Joseph.

We in the Association, are ourselves honoured, when we pay tribute to our dear friend Dr Charles Roderick Thomson.

TTMA Honours Ceremony held at the Hilton Hotel on 7th May, 1988

Laudatory Oration for Dr Martin Sampath by Dr Roderick Thomson

It is with a feeling of great honour that, on behalf of the Medical Association, I introduce, for the benefit of our newer members and our guests, a son of our southern soil, a doctor who was born at the San Fernando hospital, and years later served that same institution with distinction as one of its medical officers. I speak of Dr Martin Sylvanus Sampath, the son of the late Francis Sampath and Amelia Sampath.

Martin received his early education at Naparima College, San Fernando, and St Mary's College, Port of Spain. He then proceeded to the Imperial College of Tropical Agriculture, graduating in 1939 with the DICTA. He was a columnist in this field for the *Sunday Guardian* for three years, writing over one hundred and fifty articles under the pen name 'Agricola'. In the early days of World War II, he served as technologist for the Food Control Department of the Government of Trinidad and Tobago. His book *Food Crops and How to Grow Them* was published in 1941. He was also joint editor of the *Minerva Review*, the *Observer*, and *Why Not* magazines.

In 1942, he went to McGill University, Canada, obtaining his B.Sc. degree in 1944. He then proceeded to Leeds University, England, and graduated MB, Ch.B in 1950. As an undergraduate, he was editor of the university magazine the *Gryphon*.

On his return to Trinidad, he worked at the San Fernando hospital from 1950 to 1954, after which he did postgraduate studies at the Institute of Ophthalmology, obtaining the Diploma in Ophthalmology in 1957.

Martin is a past president of the Association, and has been a member of the Council for as long as most of us can remember, and his witticisms and clever turns of phrase, during his famous votes of thanks at our meetings, are legend and a source of inspiration for the young aspiring orators in our membership.

In addition to his many articles on agriculture, politics and economics in the lay press, and his publications on sociological topics, he has been the author of many papers published in medical journals. He has served on many special committees of the Association, and has been the Association's representative on the Board of the Institute of Marine Affairs, and its delegate at medical conferences abroad.

A man of many parts, to which the size of his family attests – six boys and three girls – Martin is a keen politician, and has been involved in party politics since its inception in Trinidad and Tobago. He has been a candidate for the PNM, the DAC and a founding member of the National Alliance for Reconstruction, which party now forms the Government of this Country.

He is a keen photographer, an aficionado of steel band and calypso, and has been chairman of a recording company which has published local music, including many of our local calypso and steel band gems.   He is at present Chairman of the Agricultural Development Bank, Deputy Chairman of Caroni Ltd, a member of the State Enterprises Review Committee, and President of the Wildlife Breeders and Farmers Association.

He has always had kind words of advice and encouragement for our younger members, and has always advocated the giving of responsibilities to new entrants.

He was awarded the Association's Scroll of Honour several years ago, and it is with pride that we now salute this eminent colleague as we invite him to accept the highest award that the Medical Association offers: the gold medal of honour.

Oration for
Dr Percival Harnarayan

*Laudatory oration by Dr Martin Sampath at the Honours Function,
held at the Texaco Club, Pointe-a-Pierre on 12th February, 1981*

Mr Percival Harnarayan MB, BS, LRCP, MRCS, FRCS FRCOG,
Specialist Medical Officer, Senior Obstetrician and Gynaecologist,
(General Hospital, San Fernando), Hospital Medical Director; born
May 4th, 1924, son of Samuel McLean Harnarayan and Ellen
Harnarayan; married Pearl Indar; educated at Naparima College, St
Mary's College, King's College, London, Westminster School of
Medicine, Royal Postgraduate School, London University, Royal
College of England and Edinburgh, Cytology Department of
Hammersmith Hospital; President of the Medical Board of Trinidad
and Tobago, and President of the Trinidad and Tobago Medical
Association.

These bald statements – a quotation from the *Who's Who in
Trinidad and Tobago* – provide but a silhouette of the person on whom
we today bestow the highest honour which the Medical Association
can offer. But, in order to appreciate the full and true significance of
this event, in 1981, we ought to remind ourselves that achievement
does not occur in isolation, but amidst the stresses and strains of an
imperfect society in perpetual labour, which has spawned as many
failures as she has produced achievers, and as many monsters as she
has saints. To bring credit to himself, his family, his Association and
to the very society which gave him birth and moulded his personality,
is achievement indeed.

When he was thirteen years old, he was in the geographical centre
of so-called oil riots, during which a policeman was burned to death
and several workers injured, within breathing distance of his
residence. The trade union movement was actively challenging the

colonial exploitation of our resources. In Fyzabad, oil had already replaced agriculture – principally cocoa – as king of the economy, yet Percy's family, with an innate love for the soil held on to their agricultural lands.

I first met Percy on a cold Christmas night in London. The German V2s were still dropping on that city. I was impressed by his dignified bearing – but perhaps it was only the deference of the medical student who was about to sit his 2nd MB towards one who had just overcome that hurdle!

But it was at the Colonial Hospital, San Fernando, that, as fellow Grade 'C' officer, he earned my respect and admiration. When he joined us it increased our strength from three to four. Our camaraderie and co-operation were as close to perfect as one could expect. We fought many battles together with the establishment. [Note: At this point of my address I related some of the incidents described in the earlier chapters of this book.]

As a result of our concerted representations, our first success was my appointment to act as DMO at Siparia. Dr Harnarayan followed me there, and on his return to the hospital succeeded me as doctor in charge of the Maternity Department. We did emergency D&Cs in the ward with screens around the bed, because the usual waiting period for the general surgeon in the operating theatre was about twenty-four hours.

I remember Dr Harnarayan meeting me at the door of the ward after I had done a Caesarean there. The mother had died suddenly during her first stage of labour. I had tried to resuscitate her with the primitive means at our disposal, but after the delay, little Julius Caesar was also unfortunately dead.

Improvements were rapid after Percy took over. The Southern Division of the Trinidad and Tobago Branch of the British Medical Association, as we then were, was very active. We had regular fortnightly clinical sessions, and my uncle Dr Shadrack Sampath, former President of the Association and a sort of benevolent godfather to all the young doctors, started an innovation: he invited all to have the Christmas session at his home, with drinks and a substantial buffet dinner. At one of these, Percy, in charge of Maternity, read a paper on his observations in Toxaemia of Pregnancy. He was warmly commended by all the senior doctors and Dr Halsey McShine, senior surgeon, correctly predicted an eminent career for Dr Harnarayan.

One of Percy's other early papers, delivered at the library of the Port of Spain Hospital, was on the subject of a National Health Plan, thus illustrating his interest and activity in the broader aspects of medical care.

While Percy did Obstetrics and Gynaecology, and I went into Ophthalmology, we still often spoke the same language: for example, we would both appreciate the fundus, and we would both have to wait for dilation – he of the parent, I of the pupil. It would not have surprised me if, at some time while at the eye clinic, I should have been asked to see some patient of his by mistake, with a letter from a general practitioner as follows: "Dear doctor, could you kindly examine and treat Mrs Jane Doe who complains that she hasn't seen anything for three months".

Percy's services to the medical board and to the Association are well known. Our present constitution is largely the result of his perseverance and acumen. His medico-legal knowledge and organisational skill have helped the Association in unbounded measure.

His practical knowledge in agriculture has been unflagging, indeed we often smile knowingly – when we do not laugh outright – every time a high sounding official pronouncement is made regarding the sugar industry, food production, family farms, the end of petroleum and so on. Percy and I had discussed these things for the past twenty-five years, and it is perhaps significant that events have now turned full circle, and the situation at Charlie King Junction in Fyzabad is again threatening the society.

We live in a society which is becoming increasingly mercenary, in which drug firms with whom we have dealt for three decades are now charging us interest on a thirty day old account, and a government which has US$6 billion of our money in United States banks, languishing and deteriorating through inflation, yet sends tax collectors to harass us in our homes. Even in this atmosphere, Dr Harnarayan has not made the earning of fees the primary motive of his profession. The patients whom I send to him all attest to his interest in their welfare as above and beyond the fees they pay.

He has walked at Kings, but kept the common touch.

Like Dr Carl Lee, the first recipient of our Gold Medal, Percy has been President, but has again accepted to serve as an officer. Carl as Treasurer and Percy as Public Relations Officer. It is significant that this officer is the only person authorised to make public statements on behalf of the Association, without prior consultation with the other officers. Percy Harnarayan is obviously eminently qualified for this responsibility.

May he be granted many, many more years of health and strength, and bring greater happiness to himself, his family, the Association and to the society which has produced him.

Oration for
Dr Roma Anita Joseph-Thomson

Laudatory oration by Dr Martin Sampath on 19th March, 1994,
at Soong's Great Wall Restaurant, San Fernando

It is an honour and a privilege for me to deliver these laudatory comments regarding our sister Roma. My pleasure is enhanced by the fact that not only is she my sister in the medical fraternity – and sorority – but she is also my den sister! Her illustrious father, Roy Joseph, before he became Mayor of San Fernando, Member of the Legislative Council, our Colony's first Minister of Education, and a member of the Parliament of the Federation of the West Indies, was my wolf cub-scout master – the father of the 5th Naparima wolf cub pack, so to speak. This was, of course, before he met Roma's mother, Dolly, daughter of an outstanding Prince of Wales Street family.

Roma is being honoured tonight for her outstanding contributions to our Association, to medicine and to our wider society, but her successes and contributions began long before this. She was born in San Fernando, and received her primary education at the San Fernando Government School. At the age of twelve, she went abroad and was enrolled at Our Lady's Convent, Oxford, and on completion of her secondary education she attended the Technical College in that City for her pre-medical science studies, then the Royal College of Surgeons, Dublin, for her medical degree.

Even at secondary school, her present qualities of service and leadership were evident: she was Prefect of her House and Head Girl of her school. She gained certificates in music, numerous prizes for deportment and elocution, and the coveted prize for *esprit de corps*. Those who now hear her expressive and melodious voice, will not be surprised to learn that she was a member of the choir which competed successfully at the London Festival and elsewhere with performances of Handel's *Messiah* and *Hiawatha.*

In 1967, she received the LRCPI, LRCSI and LM from the Royal College, then worked as a house officer at the St Lawrence's and Richmond Hospital, Dublin, in Neurology and Neurosurgery.

In 1968, she was appointed house surgeon in Neurosurgery at the San Fernando, Trinidad hospital – the hospital which her late father insisted should be in San Fernando.

In 1974, she was promoted to registrar in Neurosurgery, and when her boss, the consultant neurosurgeon, resigned, she was *ipso facto* head of that department, and her diagnostic acumen, her skill, her courage, her dedication and her amiable temperament caused her to be consulted by all the other firms faced with a possible neurological problem.

During this period, she regularly travelled the perilous route between the northern and southern capitals in order to assist Dr Sam Ghouralal at operations on the more difficult cases referred to the Port of Spain facilities. During one of these journeys in the line of duty, she sustained a severe injury to her cervical spine, for which she underwent critical spinal surgery. The resulting disability made it very difficult for her to look directly downwards at the operating table. Providentially, it made her look upwards to what is undoubtedly the highest branch of medicine – psychiatry – the study of the human mind. Judging by her successes in this field, it is clear that neurosurgery's loss was psychiatry's gain!

In 1976, she married Dr Roderick Thomson, medical officer at Pointe-a-Pierre, and although she lived there, she continued her work at San Fernando. She had been offered government scholarships in both neurosurgery and psychiatry towards higher qualifications, but she declined these offers, preferring to stay at home with her family and continue in her post as registrar. During her stint in neurosurgery she, in conjunction with Dr Thomas McKenzie, published research papers in the prestigious *Journal of Neurology, Neurosurgery and Psychiatry,* in 1970, and in the *Journal of the Royal College of Surgeons,* Edinburgh, in 1972.

Anyone who has witnessed her host of extra-curricular activities in Trinidad will not be surprised to learn that, while in England, she was secretary of her students' union, and later president. She represented

Ireland at the UNESCO sponsored conference in Geneva in 1963. She was on the debating team at the TIMES debate in Ireland. She won the Bronze, Silver and later the Gold medal in elocution and Drama, in 1957, and, in 1958, the Diploma in Verse Speaking, and, in 1959, the Bronze medal in acting from the London Academy of Music and Dramatic Art.

In Trinidad, she was a member of our Council, Chairman of the Southern Branch, and in 1987, our President. She presided over the organisation of our nation's first renal transplants, and has represented our Association at conferences in Trinidad and Jamaica and at certain proceedings at the UWI Faculty of Medicine. Because of her capabilities as a moderator, she is systematically invited to preside at clinical meetings, especially those involving visiting dignitaries.

She is an active member of the Soroptimist Club in San Fernando, an executive member since 1982, and president for 1987 and 1988. She was chairman of its civil action committee, in 1989, and has represented the club in Jamaica and Barbados.

Roma is a member of the important National Council on Alcoholism and Substance Abuse, and has taken special courses at the Caribbean Institute in St Thomas.

She has a finely honed and discriminatory taste in literature, antique silver, music (shared by her husband), the arts, gourmet cuisine and wine – the imbibing variety.

Although she has chosen not to have children of her own, at least for the present – she is a devoted and affectionate mother to her three stepchildren, conveniently provided for her by her dear husband Roderick. Such devotion and affection are obviously fully reciprocated by all the members of her family, colleagues and friends.

Based on all that I have said, certain deductions and guidelines of a general nature seem to emerge.

(1) Genetic inheritance and cultural inheritance can combine to produce excellence of the highest order.

(2) Nationalism and a commendable pride in our Asian and African genetic and cultural heritage must not blind us to the real value of our European cultural inheritance which is an inescapably potent part of our history.

(3) There are, among us, persons who, despite the blandishments of metropolitan prestige and financial gain, are strong enough

to reverse the so-called 'brain drain' and enrich our society with their exceptional skills.

One of her admirers says of her, "Roma is an eminent representative of that disappearing class of cultured and truly educated doctors. She is a person of deep, religious conviction who measures all her professional activities by the high standards of ethics and moral principles that she has set for herself. Her working colleagues regard her as selfless in her efforts to mitigate suffering, and her patients adulate her and respond sensitively to her ministrations."

Roma, we all love you for the person you are. We admire you for your accomplishments, and we thank and honour you for your contributions to our nation.

A Note on the Following Chapters

In the Senate, the upper house of parliament in our country, my official portfolios were Agriculture and Medicine, but all Senators, whatever their special interests or qualifications, were encouraged to contribute to debates on any topic on which they thought they could make constructive comments.   I took full advantage of this convention. For the purposes of this book, however, I include a few of those which have a bearing on medical matters, reproduced from the Hansard transcript.

Readers will doubtless observe that the style is largely conversational – often unnecessarily verbose and repetitive. Unlike so many of our illustrious colleagues in parliament, some of us spoke from notes, instead of reading out a prepared essay – the latter is not permitted by the rules of parliament, but this is generally observed only in the breach.

The Dangerous Drugs Bill

BS 91.08.27:2.15 p.m.

Mr President, I feel deeply privileged to be able to speak on this extremely important Bill, at this stage in the development of our country. It is a country which at present is suffering from increasing crime and from an increasing lack of responsibility on the part of a great many individuals and a great many agencies. We must understand that drug trafficking and the use of these dangerous drugs are at the root of a great many of the crimes which exist in the country. So that, unlike my honourable friend, the last speaker, I feel that we must strike at the root of this pernicious tree before we can solve a great many of the crimes that exist today

In my contribution, I hope to show how these various things interact, and how they tie up with drug trafficking and the use of dangerous drugs. I think this Senate is honoured to have so many brilliant forensic minds. Unfortunately, the same is not true about the composition of the medical side or the agricultural side of the Senate. In my contribution, I hope to make up for that glaring deficiency. I have made a few notes, and very briefly I will give a skeleton of what I propose to say this afternoon.

First, I want to record my regrets that my medical colleagues, temporary senators Bharat and Sealey, are not here this evening, because they told me that they had prepared to speak on this Bill. It is left to me to deal with the medical side.

I want to talk about the changing attitudes in Trinidad and Tobago with reference to marijuana and cocaine which are two of the most dangerous drugs here, for geographical reasons. Opium, heroin and morphine have found their way in the old world because they are more prevalent there, and marijuana and cocaine in the new world because the source of these plants has been indigenous to South America and the West.

I shall refer to what some of our scientists said until recently, about these two drugs, and the attitude that they had, very, very recently, in this country. I will go on to talk a little bit more about society and the behaviour of people, and then I shall talk about the actual taxonomy of these plants, that is to say, the classification of the plants, insofar as the production of marijuana and cocaine is concerned. Next, I will say a few words about police powers and their deficiencies, then about penalties, whether they are too stiff or too mild, and then, in order that I shall bring honourable senators of this House face to face with the actual problem of addiction, I shall give two case histories with which I myself have dealt personally and which brought me face to face, among other cases, with the problem of addiction and how it affects the parents and the people around them. Then I shall talk about preventive measures and what this Government has been doing, then the question of treatment and the overloaded facilities and then, finally, the question of curtailment of liberties and how we should react to, what appears to be certain curtailment of the liberties of the citizens in order to deal with this problem.

Now with the changing conditions in the culture of the country, with reference to cocaine and marijuana, I think everybody knows that, not so long ago, it was possible to buy marijuana in the shops openly. There were signs saying: "Licensed to sell Ganja by Retail", and people smoked it, and they relaxed and there was no problem. There was very little addiction, if any, and it never affected society. Now, as far as cocaine is concerned, things were a little different. Cocaine has been known for a long time medically. It has been used as a surface anaesthetic, a contact anaesthetic for mucosal tissue, for example, the eye, and for operations done on the surface of the eye. It has been used in very small injections for the extraction of teeth, and it has had its dangers. One thing that happened to a very senior colleague of mine, an ophthalmologist, who wanted to do a nerve block on a patient's eye, was that instead of injecting one of the synthetic drugs, like procaine, provocaine or novocaine into the back of the eye to deaden the nerve, the nurse handed him a vial of cocaine which he injected, the patient died from an overdose of cocaine, and he had to pay considerable damages.

Now, to show you how scientists find it difficult to foresee what can happen to some of the drugs that are in existence, I want to quote from a book. The book is called *Useful and Ornamental Plants of Trinidad and Tobago*, by R.O. Williams and, his son, R.O. Williams Jnr. In the 1969 edition – you see it is very recent, only 1969 – he describes marijuana in the following terms: "Cannabis sativa: Family Moraceae, Hemp, Ganjah. An erect, annual herb three to twelve feet high, cultivated in cool climates for its fibre and oilseed. Leaves of three to seven long narrow leaflets" and so on, "the flowers" and all that, and he says, "Grown in the tropics, a resin is produced, especially in the flower tops of female plants which when dried has an intoxicating, narcotic effect when smoked. The cultivation of this plant is prohibited in the colony."

Even then, the cultivation of this plant was prohibited in the colony, and that is all he says. The question of addiction is not raised.

Now, let us look at what he said about the plant that produces cocaine: "Erythroxolon novo-granatense. Family: Erythroxylaceae, coca, cocaine plant. A shrub with light green oval leaves, short spikes of small white flowers succeeded by small red fruits". (Incidentally, this is how it gets its name Erythroxylum. Erythrocyte is a red blood cell. Erythros means red.)

"The value of the plant became known because it was used by the Indians of Peru and Bolivia, the leaves, chewed with lime or infused like tea increasing the nervous energy and endurance and lessening fatigue". Now, listen to this, "It makes a good hedge"!

This is all he has to say about the cocaine plant. Even at that time, 1969, there was no law about not growing this particular plant. So you see how things have changed between then and now.

Many people who helped him with this, like Professor Cheeseman, who was my Professor at the Imperial College of Tropical Agriculture, Dr Pound, who did research on cocoa, F.M. Bain and so on – I knew these gentlemen very well – not a word about addiction. It shows what the attitude of even our scientists was to the drugs in those days. "Why has this become a problem in the country today?" one asks. It is a terrible problem. Why did it happen? Now, when doctors knew that cocaine was dangerous, they started using the synthetic substances which had a cocaine-like effect on anaesthesia, but the question still arises: why is it that doctors still have a great deal of difficulty with some of these dangerous drugs, not only these two but other dangerous drugs? When I speak about the patient I had, who became addicted because doctors gave him one of these dangerous drugs, you will understand how deeply this problem is located.

Why is it that these drugs have become so terrible? An analogy, I believe, that came across my mind, was the locust, the simple locust. You know, the biology of small animals is very similar to that of large animals. I think Professor Spence will be able to confirm this. When the locust is in its solitary phase, it is physically harmless. It eats a few plants, does not kill any, and that is all right. You can have thousands of locusts in the solitary phase, but then you get the gregarious phase where they all get together, and the psychology and physiology change to the point where they become a major menace to crops all over the world. They march like an army, and just destroy things.

So, it does appear that moving from a rural and a scattered environment into urban areas, where they are crowded and where there is stress of one kind or another, does lead people to become addicts on the same drugs that were available when they lived in more scattered areas. You see, this has happened all over the world. It happened in the metropolitan areas first of all. It has now spread to the so-called third world countries, we who seem to ape the worst vices of the metropolitan areas without following the virtues of better production and higher skills and so on. We, in the third world countries, seem to suffer from that particular vice. That seems to be an explanation. It is not the only explanation, but it seems to be one.

Now, Mr President, this thing is so important, the actual source of cocaine which is the major peril in this country, that we in the Senate have always been on the cutting edge of science and technology. We were at the cutting edge of this in the Domestic Violence Bill, also in the Telecommunications Bill. Things that are to develop in the future, we have already thought about here, and have provisions for. The same thing is happening now with this Dangerous Drugs Bill. I will tell you exactly where I am coming from in that respect.

Some of you may have seen a copy of this tentative amendment, which has been circulated, having to do with the definition of the coca plant, and, also, I am suggesting a new definition of the word 'plant', and this is what I am talking about – the cutting edge of technology. What alerted me to this was a small typographical error on page two of the definitions. The definition of 'coca plant', according to the Bill before us: "means a plant of the genus Erythroxylaceae, from which cocaine can be extracted".

They referred to 'genus Erythroxylaceae'. Now any taxonomist or botanist will realise that 'erythroxylaceae' is the name of a family. The genus is 'Erythroxylum', having been alerted to this I read up a little more about the source of cocaine and I was not happy about it, so I telephoned Dr Seaforth who is an expert on the production of chemicals and medicines by plants. (He wrote a book called *Medicinal Plants of Trinidad and Tobago*.) I telephoned him, and asked him about this; I said, "Dr Seaforth, are there any other members of this family which produce cocaine?" He said, "Well I will look up my references." He is an expert in this field and he knows where to look. He telephoned me the next morning, and he gave me some very interesting information. He said to me, "You know, Dr Sampath, the two plants that are cultivated, from which cocaine is extracted, are Erythroxylum coca and Erythroxylum novogranatense. These two produce cocaine in commercial quantities, but there are two wild species in Venezuela just next door: Erythroxylum recurrens and Erythroxylum steyermarkii which produce just as much cocaine."

These are not yet cultivated, but believe you me, Mr President, these barons who are making the money, you can bet your bottom dollar that they are investigating all the plants that can produce cocaine and they are going to do it. And these two plants are just next door in Venezuela. So my point here is tentative, but when you have this information, it will be up to us in the Senate to devise wording which will ensure that none of these plants can come into this country, and that the law will protect us from the introduction of these plants.

Now, again, we are at the cutting edge of science and technology, and we must be aware that the word 'plant' must be defined even further, because a 'plant' is a plant with roots, stems, leaves and flowers: that is the dictionary definition of a plant. But these days, it is possible to have genetic material and gene transplants. Again, you can rest assured that these drug barons, and those who assist in the cultivation of the cocaine and related plants, are making sure that they will be able to get tissue, and introduce some of these deadly genes into other species. So, we must widen the definition of 'plant' to include genetic materials, such as plant cell tissue or scion material.

You know, the 'scion' is the part which you graft on to another plant. You can take a sour orange and graft on a grapefruit and get grapefruit. Everybody knows about this. So we have to guard against all this, so it is for the Senate and the legal minds among us to draft the wording which will make it impossible for any of these people to benefit from a little deficiency in this bill.

I have just discussed the taxonomy of the toxicology, that is to say the classification of plants and the poisons they produce.

Now, the question of police powers has been hinted at. This is one of the weakest areas in our entire society, and it has been so since colonial times. Fortunately, we have people, now in the ministry, looking after this, who are making sure that the recruitment of new police officers is such that the attitude towards their work and towards their citizens is much more healthy than it has been in the past. It is not going to be easy. There are still 'black sheep' in the police service, among the higher echelons and lower echelons, as there are in any other profession, among doctors, lawyers, businessmen, everywhere. But we are trying our best to see that the police do their work properly. It is certainly weak, perhaps the weakest link in everything, in all the laws that we pass here.

The question of penalties: are the penalties too stiff? In the East, they execute a man if he is found with a certain amount of drugs. The penalties are not stiff at all. I think the penalties are perhaps too mild, if anything, when you think about the damage that these drug traffickers and drug barons do.

Now I would like to relate to you two case histories. They are very sad case histories, but I want to take away from your minds that drug addiction is a question of statistics, of reading in the papers what happens to a person in Sangre Grande or a person in San Fernando, it is a very real thing. When I read these, you will see. I want to bring you face to face with the addict, face to face with what his family faces, what his friends face, what his brothers and sisters face.

The first is a young man, of about thirty-five years, who drives big trucks belonging to a contractor - very heavy vehicles. I have correspondence here, between myself and the Chief Medical Officer, concerning this gentleman. As a matter of fact, I had to protect myself, because at one time it was felt that I was making him an addict. From this correspondence, you will see the problem of not only the man, but the lengths to which addicts can go, and the danger

222

to the doctor who might be treating these addicts. This has a bearing on what my honourable colleague, Senator Maharaj, has told you about doctors using drugs for treating these addicts. It is a very complicated thing. Let me start and read the correspondence.

The first letter I got was from the Chief Medical Officer stamped CONFIDENTIAL in red, dated 1st June, 1979.

Dear Dr Sampath, During recent inspections of records of narcotic drugs at pharmacies, officers of the drug inspectorate, Ministry of Health, have discovered that considerable quantities of narcotics drugs, namely Pethidine, have been prescribed for a patient, Mr Hal (Note: In my contribution, in the interest of confidentiality I used only the last syllable of the patient's surname), of Erin Road, Siparia. Prescriptions, alleged to be signed by you, have been produced both at King's Pharmacy, Cipero Street, San Fernando, and at Garcia's Pharmacy, Fyzabad Road, Guapo. During January to February 1978, Mr Hal received some 268 x 50 mgs Pethidine tablets. I should be grateful to have information from you on this, and the medical reasons for prescribing large quantities of narcotics for this patient. Naturally, your explanation will be treated with the greatest confidence.

My reply dated 18th June.

"Dear doctor [name mentioned], I thank you for your letter of 1st June. This patient suffers from a very painful gastrointestinal condition, and for many years has been treated by other doctors at the General Hospital, San Fernando, with narcotics, to which he has developed considerable tolerance. He has been having repeated injections of narcotics, and I have got out of bed at night on several occasions, sometimes twice the same night, in June, 1977. I am pleased to say that he has been weaned off injections. At least I have not given him an injection for nearly a year, and he is gradually being transferred to Sosegon tablets.

Now if you look at the schedule attached to this Bill, you will see drugs related to Sosegon are also listed here, for a very good reason. Sosegon is, incidentally, a synthetic drug which has some of the qualities of morphine and some of the qualities of amphetamine.

The next letter is in June, 1979:

Thank you for your letter of 18th June. I will ask you to provide us with another report. Meanwhile, I am of the view that he will have to be considered an addict.

I then read parts of the exchange of several letters between us. It appears that many more prescriptions were being discovered at pharmacies, allegedly signed by me and having my rubber stamp on them. In desperation, in 1981, I asked to see the prescriptions. The fraud squad visited me with the prescriptions, and lo and behold, none of the signatures were mine, they carried my rubber stamp, and some of the letterheads were photostats. So, this unfortunate young man, driven by his addiction was forging my prescriptions and signature, and getting the Pethidine from a variety of pharmacies.

This story has a very sad ending. The fraud squad got on to him. I do not know what happened; I believe that they wanted to arrest him. He committed suicide by drinking the weedkiller called Gramoxone. It shows, you see, the deficiency in everything, the deficiency in the way we think about victims. Drug addicts are not criminals, they are victims. The criminals are the pushers, the criminals are the traffickers, and the criminals are the drug barons.

Why do some people become addicted to anything, to cigarettes, to caffeine? There is something in the personality of the human being which is not 100% flawless; some of us are weaker, some are frailer in some respects; some of us are a little bit schizophrenic. However, these people do not get heart attacks simply because they are schizophrenic; I have never heard of a myocardial infarct in a schizophrenic in my life; they protect themselves from stress by taking themselves away from stress. So, you see, being a little bit different and being frail sometimes is a protection for the person, but unfortunately when you have substances readily available for them they take a step in the wrong direction.

If it is cigarettes, nothing is wrong with that. Some of my best friends are nicotine addicts. Some of them are in the Senate today. Whenever they smoke during committee stages, I move a little away from them because I do not want to be addicted to nicotine. So, there is nothing wrong, really, with being frail or being weak.

I will now read the case history of the second person because it is important.

Now, this person became addicted to cocaine, and he went through all the stages. He is about thirty years old now. I attended to his mother when she was pregnant with him. From the day she became pregnant I attended to her, right through. She had a very normal pregnancy, with one exception: she was one month overdue. I try to look for reasons, reasons in the environment or in the personality, as to why he might be addicted, and so I paid particular attention to this young man. I know him very well. When I was delivering him, I had to give his mother an injection to contract her uterus which had stopped contracting, so that he could emerge. He would have died before he was born if I hadn't done so. He was a normal, charming child. The only thing I could see wrong with him as he grew up was that he liked the ladies very much and I always joked with his mother: "You know why he likes the ladies? Because he stayed inside you too long." But you see, you can joke about certain things, but it became very serious with him after a time, Mr President.

He went to one of the prestige schools in San Fernando. He got six O-levels and, at that time, he started with alcohol, tobacco, marijuana, so he did not finish his A-levels, but got married when he was twenty, and now has two charming children, a boy and a girl aged nine and eight respectively.

He got a job as a trainee-supervisor in one of the oilfields, and made tremendous progress. He won snooker tournaments and so on: the trophies are in the house. Then, he started cocaine while he was working for this company, and that changed him completely. I could not detect anything different in his personality, except this immense charm, when he was growing up. I treated him for nephritis, chicken pox, measles, mumps. He went through all these things, and came out shining.

But with cocaine, he changed. He started absenting himself from work. His father and mother would drop him off at the bus station to go to work, and they would find him skulking in the house in the morning. Having been dropped, he went and got his cocaine and came back. Then he started beating his wife.

You see, if people ask, "Why are you rushing these Bills?" my response is that we are not rushing them. The fact is that there are things in society which need to be changed. Society is like the human body. We have got to treat every aspect of the diseases and shortcomings in society. This ties up with the Domestic Violence Bill, so we had to get that through. Then Telecommunications, the question of monitoring, the question of knowing codes. We have to know what these drug traffickers and other people are doing. They mesh together. It is an holistic effort we are making here.

This young man started showing signs of paranoia. He had started having delusions of grandeur, that he was better than anyone else, also delusions of people taking advantage of him, delusions of persecution, blaming his parents, blaming his wife, blaming everybody.

His wife has been very faithful to him, has been very kind to him. She loves him. She married him for love, not for money. She is sticking by him all the time, no matter what he does, she sticks by him. Mr President, why does a woman love a man? I am convinced that a woman can admire a man for his strengths, but she loves him for his weaknesses. This is a case that illustrates it – she has never left him.

He started stealing. He does not call it stealing. He does not deny that he has taken those things, but he takes from his own home. He takes money from his father, mother, wife and children. The children's piggy bank is always empty, jewellery, equipment. I say 'take' because he boasts that he does not steal from anybody else, only from his family, what he feels belongs to him. But I will make another point later, (because his parents between them are worth several million dollars): the contrast between that and the person who does not have anything. I shall return to this a little later when I come to deal with society and other things.

He took lamps, electric and ornamental, emergency pitch-oil, light bulbs, electric extension cords, batteries, barbed wire – eight rolls, dozens of twenty foot lengths of PVC pipes, the car radio, welding rods, an electric fan, and also a hundred dollar glass fish tank. He steals clothing, his own trousers, shirts, socks, shoes, T-shirts, underwear, his children's clothes, dozens of rolls of toilet paper, soap, soap powder, toothpaste. He takes these things, and exchanges them for a ten-dollar cocaine rock which he puts in a cigarette and lights up. He takes foodstuffs from the kitchen, dozens of tins of condensed milk, twenty-four cartons of sta-fresh milk, cartons of butter. When his mother thinks that there is something there to cook, it is not there. It sounds funny, you know, but it is tragic.

One day, his mother told me that she took out a leg of lamb from the freezer, had it there to defrost for the Sunday's lunch. He came in about nine o'clock, and she said to him, "Now, are you going out again?" because his habit was to come in and then sneak out and go and take his cocaine. He said no, he was going to bed. Suddenly, she heard something. She got up and looked, and the leg of lamb was gone. He had taken this, opened the door, and gone out to exchange it, presumably for two cocaine rocks.

I see the Minister of External Affairs smiling. It can be funny, you know. In fact if you did not think it funny, you would cry.

Now, when there was nothing in the house that he could be entrusted with, his parents locked the house, and said, "Now, look here, you have got to sleep in the garage, if you come in here, you will steal everything we have." What does he do? He started stealing the plants that she had around, mango plants, and sold them. He started digging up plants from the yard, and selling them. He is very clever. He can pick the locks of the car, and comes in when he wants to, listens around at conversations in the house and so on. The effect on his family is tragic. Imagine how his father, mother, wife and children are suffering. Think of the anguish that these people have when they know that this person, a person she gave birth to, that she trained, sent to school, and all of that, has dropped to that level. Just think of it. I do not mind telling you when he started getting on and shouting at everybody and all that, at one time she said, "Look, if I had a gun, I would shoot him."

This is the reality of the addict, Mr President. This is why we must stop these drugs from coming into the country. We must do it because of thousands and thousands of young people, men and women – when a young woman is addicted and has nothing more to sell, you know, she sells herself. This is what we are facing.

So let us not pussy-foot about this. Let us not talk about, "this is useless, unless we do the other thing before passing this law". Is anyone suggesting that this Parliament should now shut down and stop passing laws because we do not have infrastructure for dealing with these things? It is ridiculous, Mr President. I do not know what to say when I hear people saying that. Do they not understand that these drugs are at the root of so many crimes that we have? We trim a branch here, we trim a branch there, we catch a thief here, we get a motor car there and so on, but if the root of the thing is not dealt with, if these drug barons are not brought to heel, if their property is not confiscated and used for the purposes for which provision is made in this Bill, we will never solve the problems of the country.

So, let us be very careful when we try to delay this Bill for another three years. I am not surprised, Mr President, that certain people on this side of the house hinted that the reason why there was delay was because there were perhaps people on some other side or in some other place, who were in league with drug barons. I am not surprised. People can get emotional and think that kind of thing. But I am not saying so, what I am saying is that that is the danger if we delay this Bill any further.

These poor children of this person, this patient of mine that I am talking about, this boy and this girl, their nerves have gone. This poor little fellow starts wheezing whenever the father starts getting on. He wets his bed when these things happen. Is he going to be a victim too when he gets older?[16] What do you think he will be? What are the chances of his not becoming an addict and following in his father's footsteps? These thousands of young people in the country must be helped, and there is provision in this Bill to the effect that when property and money are seized, confiscated, from these drug barons and traffickers, they will be used for the rehabilitation of these addicts.

This young man that I am talking about: I referred him to a psychiatrist; he went up to Caura. He stayed there for two months. He came back to his family and apparently everything was all right, until he started working again. This urge is so great, this urge for cocaine is something which sometimes I wish I could experience, so that I could tell you what it feels like; but, of course, one shot can get you addicted, so I do not experiment with it. But what they tell me is that the pleasure one derives from smoking cocaine is immensely greater than anything else. They tell me that it is greater than smoking a cigarette after you have been deprived, or slaking your

---

[16] With his superior intelligence and tremendous willpower and now residing in the USA, he has won a Certificate of Achievement in the Drug Abuse Resistance Programme and the award by the President of the United States for 'Outstanding Academic Achievement in 1995'. A magnificent future awaits him. And will the son reform the father?

thirst after a football game. It is even ten times more pleasurable than sexual intercourse.

Now, you see, such intense pleasure means the urge is tremendous, and that is why people say, 'Once a cocaine addict, always an addict'. The withdrawal symptoms are such that the addicts are a menace to themselves and other people.

Now, I want to talk about the poor person. Unlike the rich addict, the poor person goes and steals from strangers, and ends up in jail. There are thousands of such persons in jail today.

Mr President, I think I have said enough. I want to exhort this honourable house, there are amendments to be made, make the amendments, but in the final analysis, Mr President, through you, may I say to my colleagues here, please, for the sake of your children – these two people could be your children, they could be the children of any one of us – we must not wait too much longer. Procrastination is the thief of many things, especially of time, and let it not be the thief of this particular Bill.

So for the sake of all our children, please pass this Bill quickly and unanimously.

(Author's Note: I have omitted several paragraphs from the original transcript which appeared, on re-reading to be unnecessarily repetitive. While such repetition may have some value as emphasis in verbal communication, it would be merely a waste of print, paper and a reader's time and patience!)

Crime and Cocaine

The following article was published in Newsday *of 29th July, and* Guardian *of 24th August, 1994*

It has been estimated that 80% of thefts, murders and other crimes of violence are drug related. What this means is that most of the items stolen are sold in order to purchase cocaine. The stolen goods are disposed of, for a small fraction of their true market value: a three hundred dollar car radio, for example, will fetch $60 – the price of six rocks of crack cocaine; a $40 leg of lamb will be eagerly sold by an addict for $20; and a $30 orchid plant in flower will be given away for a single rock.

In his withdrawal phase, when the craving is intense, the addict may be uncontrollably maniacal, and may maim or kill for the price of a single dose.

The cocaine addict, before the establishment of his addiction often has a paranoid personality: he harbours a sense of grievance against his parents, his siblings and his society, especially those members whom he perceives to be his superiors by virtue of education, wealth, class or skin colour. He regards these persons as his oppressors, responsible for his lowly station in life. This paranoia is heightened by his use of cocaine, and his thefts and assaults – especially including his sexual assaults, when they are performed, regarded by him as a means of physical and psychological revenge on his imagined oppressors, and as a 'logical' (to him) means of financial redress.

A rock of crack cocaine costs twenty cents to produce. The retail price in 1994 is $10. (In 1992 it was $5). When shipments are seized (after a tip-off of sometimes questionable origin), the price tends to increase. The profits, gained by the manufacturers, drug barons, transporters, agents and pushers are enormous, even if one includes, as expenses, the monies paid for police protection and to those propagandists who strive assiduously to keep the trade as illegal as possible. Their final clients – the consuming addicts and their victims, we, the rest of society – are the ones who pay the price.

The list of beneficiaries of this illegal drug trade would include, not only the barons and their accomplices, but also the manufacturers and businessmen who quite legitimately replace stolen or vandalised goods, the doctors who humanely treat the injured persons for their accepted fees, the lawyers who, in the completely ethical practice of their professions represent the attackers, the attacked, the thieves and their victims and of course, the minor pushers, when caught. Tragically, a benefit is also derived for the undertaker, the seamstress who is called upon to produce a black dress at short notice, and the florist and horticulturist who, in a combined effort, assist in the demonstration of sympathy to the unfortunate victim of cocaine. We must not forget that all the media also benefit: the sensation provided by all aspects of cocaine, especially any tragic consequences, are grist for their mill, and adrenalin for the circulation of their product.

In short, illegal drug trafficking is a black market which impinges on and permeates – unsuspected – our entire body politic, and is one of the hidden fuels of our economy.

Historically, the illegal cocaine trade in these last decades of the twentieth century, has its closest parallel in Prohibition, during the early decades of this same century, in the United States of America. At that time, illegal alcohol was directly and indirectly responsible for widespread violence and murderous assaults. The end of prohibition coincided with a marked reduction in corruption among the police and among government officials, since 'protection' was no longer necessary.

So what can we do about cocaine? The obvious answer is that since its illegality is largely the cause of the crime problem, let us decriminalise it, and do so as a matter of extreme urgency. I therefore recommend that the following practical steps be undertaken simultaneously:

(1) Register all cocaine addicts on a voluntary basis for a small registration fee, say $20.
(2) Set up an agency, under the aegis of the Ministry of Health and Social Services, for the free supply and distribution of cocaine to all registered addicts.

(3) Expand the existing rehabilitation centres and extend them to all regions of the country. These centres should operate under the supervision of the drug agency and could follow the admirable example of the Rebirth House in Port of Spain which emphasises agricultural (food production) and artistic activity. The agency and its centres can be financed by government subventions, private donations and the sale – and self-utilisation – of the goods produced by the rehabilitees themselves. A government subvention is fully justified, in view of the savings to government which must accrue as a result of the removal of potential cocaine related crimes from our midst: the reduction of property loss, police expenses, prosecution costs, medical and legal expenditure and so on.

(4) Intensify the education of citizens of all ages regarding the dangers to body and mind of cocaine and other addictive drugs including alcohol and tobacco.

(5) Acquire and safeguard (especially from rodents[17]) all available stocks of cocaine. It will also be necessary to purchase the drug from existing suppliers, who must be allowed to operate only under licence. The market value of cocaine, as soon as it ceases to be illegal, will drop to approximately one and a half times its cost of production. Most manufacturers and drug barons will find this unprofitable by their former standards and will go out of business, as will the crime rate.

There are many who oppose decriminalisation on the grounds that, with legality, cocaine's use will spread like wildfire, especially if it were cheaply obtainable. I ask some of these critics, "If you got it free, would you use it?" The answer is invariably, "No". Most of these critics are conscientious persons, but sadly a few of them have a conscious vested interest in the illegality of the substance, and these tend to be the most vocal and influential.

The fact is, that if someone is so disposed, he or she will use cocaine whatever the legal status and whatever the cost – even if he

---

[17] When questioned about the unavailability of a substantial batch of seized cocaine as evidence, the police gave the excuse that it was eaten up by rats!

232

has to get it by violent means and it is here that an intense educational programme goes to work. At our rehabilitation centres, as a result of the openness with which the drug is handled and discussed because of its decriminalised status, it would be possible for useful experimentation to be conducted towards the 'cure' of those addicted, for example, the use of cocaine-like substitutes, skin patches and the utilisation of our abundant local cocaine producing plant, the *Erythroxylum novo-granatense* as a chewable product or as a tincture.

The crime situation in our country calls for bold, if to some, unorthodox measures. Punishment in all the forms currently being adopted is not working and will never work.

Let us proceed boldly and decriminalise this substance now.

*

There were two published disagreements with my recommendation for decriminalisation.

Mr Mardy Mohammed of Petit Valley wrote, *inter alia*:

"I can't quite understand how Dr Sampath reached the conclusion that the problem with cocaine is its illegality... Legalising of cocaine will not work because the government will have to buy the whole of Columbia to keep the addicts satisfied..."

Mr Israel B. Khan, a prominent criminal attorney of Port of Spain wrote:

"Dr Martin Sampath... advocated that in order to get rid of cocaine, we should decriminalise it..."

Both gentlemen missed the target (crime) by pot-shotting at the scaffolding (cocaine)!

The Abuse of Children

*(Abridged from the author's contribution to the debate on the
'Children's Amendment Bill',
from* Hansard, Senate: *17 September, 1991)*

Mr President, this has been a very short, straightforward Bill, and the fact that it has evoked so much intelligent discussion and so many contributions is clear evidence that Senators here identify with their children and with the children of the nation to the extent that they probably feel that our children are our only true immortality.

I am impelled to speak for two reasons: the first, is that I do not think, in spite of the excellent contributions, that we have considered sufficiently the historical perspective of the evolution of violence towards children, which in our society is most peculiar and interesting. Professor Lloyd Brathwaite, our well known and eminent sociologist, stated in one of his books that, although people in this country loved their children very much, yet, they were most brutal in chastising them. This is borne out by several other writers.

Naipaul's *Loss of El Dorado*, a historical documentary dealing with events in Trinidad at the time of Picton and the British accession, at page 385, includes the following fascinating description.

'The severe judicial whipping of children continues to be one of the solemn dramas of Trinidad backyard life. A badly beaten child is said to be 'blessed'. This is from the French 'blesser', to wound, but the word is spoken as an English word, which has the association of church, sacrament and awe. A blessing is an occasion for stillness. The blesser is handled with care by his women folk, while the mood of stillness lasts he is a man apart, fragile, touched by an unnatural and even divine frenzy. For the blessed child there is special affection and a special food of love: butter in hot sugared milk. The mood of stillness becomes a mood of sweetness. It is known that after a blessing everyone is closer. The drama that has been enacted... both in its master-slave reality and its man-child mimicry, is, of course, the drama of the plantation whip, transmuted into a dream of community.'

So, we must remember that violence towards children is something which has very deep psychological and historical roots. We must also realise that parents in a 'divine frenzy' tend to inflict punishment that is much too severe, and this is the reason for the intervention of the state.

There is another psychological factor at work here: beating can be a form of masochism – the parent identifies with the child. In beating the child, he is beating himself, and this is the origin of the phrase: 'this hurts me more than it hurts you'. It is important for a parent to have a certain insight as to why be beats his child.

Another reason why a parent may beat a child is because of the sense of guilt they may have in the pleasure of actually producing the child. This may sound far fetched to some of you, but if you project it to its extreme, say, when a parent has an unwanted child or is an unmarried mother, they may beat this child much more cruelly than they would his or her brother or sister.

Interestingly, there has been a dramatic reversal of cruel discipline since World War II: parents have become extremely tolerant of erratic children. Parents seem to think: 'Now look at what we have done: we have brought children into the world, into a society which we have made so unsuitable and so unhealthy for them.' This attitude was exacerbated after the Vietnam War.

In a lecture which I gave to the graduating class of Iere High School in Siparia, on October 25th, 1968, I said, "And now in closing, may I ask you students to understand the problems of your parents, if they do not always appear to see eye to eye with you? They have had their uncertainties, inflations and devaluations. And parents, if your children appear to be wild and rebellious at times, please remember that we as parents of this world have not provided an eminently stable or secure environment in which they must grow up. The hippies and flower people are the generations which, in infancy and early childhood were paraded in and out of air raid shelters, in an atmosphere of tension and fear of impending dissolution from nuclear attack." (That was 1968 – the height of the Cold War). "Even now, there is a twenty-four hour alert, with planes always in the sky, armed with nuclear war heads, prepared to strike the first blow. Where there is a twenty-four hour alert, there must be a corresponding twenty-four hour relaxation, and this is generously provided by the flower people who insist on constantly making love not war."

So the pendulum of violence to children has swung far out in the direction of extreme tolerance, as it has swung in other areas. In Russia, it has swung from feudalism to communism and back again reaching the point of capitalism. It will certainly come to rest somewhere in the centre of the extreme ideologies. The pendulum of violence to children may now swing the other way. Parents may now start brutalising their children, and the intervention of the state, as with these amendments, will be necessary.

Sexual Abuse of Children and Young Adults

This produces tremendous psychological damage. The actual physical damage may not be very much, and I shall deal with those aspects later.

Now, incest is an interesting subject: it is quite natural among animals, among ancient Egyptian royalty and among ancient Britons. Julius Caesar in his *De Bello Gallico* describes domestic arrangements in Britain at the time of his invasion, and found that incest was the norm. In the matriarchal society, the father and the sons lived in the same house with the mother, and all the males had sexual relations with her. I am personally disgusted with the idea of incest, but, remember that incest is a difficult thing to prove in our society, and lawyers must be very careful. Some time ago, one of our calypsonians, Lord Melody, sang a ditty called 'Shame and a Scandal in the Family' which described how this young man, who wanted to marry a certain young lady, was told by his father, "No, you cannot. She is your sister, but your mother doesn't know." This happened again with two other girls, so the dejected suitor complained to his mother who told him, "Boy, you can marry any of them. Your father is not your father but your father doesn't know!"

On the question of physical damage to a minor: there may be very little physical damage when a stepfather has relations with his grown-up stepdaughter, but the psychological damage can be profound. It can be profound from the economic standpoint as well. It can prevent the girl from forming a satisfactory relationship with someone else, and spoils her chances of getting married.

Last Tuesday, two ladies came into my office with a child. The younger lady was the daughter-in-law of the elder. Both child and mother had a very easily treatable skin infection. I noticed from the card that the child was one year old and the mother was fourteen. She was a very healthy looking, lovely and well-developed woman and I thought that the receptionist had made a mistake about her age. I asked her, "Did you have this baby when you were thirteen?"

"Oh yes," she replied.

"Is he your first child?"

"No," she told me, "I have two others." So, she had three children before she was fifteen! There was no physical damage of any kind and there was no psychological damage either, because she had a husband, protective in-laws with whom she was living and everything was hunky-dory.

It is the very opposite when a stepfather gets his stepdaughter pregnant.

We amend our laws, from time to time, so that, in repairing the damage done to our national psyche, we keep pace with modern thinking. In this way, we gradually break the shackles of the worst aspects of our unfortunate and often savage historical antecedents. These amendments let it be known formally that we have relinquished those attitudes we developed when we were unwillingly in servitude.

At the start of my presentation, I said that there were two reasons why I felt impelled to speak today: the first was the historical perspective with which I have dealt. The second reason is entirely egotistical: I wanted to have the honour of addressing this honourable Senate on the 72nd anniversary of my own birth. Today is my birthday.

Epilogue

The enormous strides made in diagnostic techniques and treatment, both medical and surgical, since the late 1940s, are phenomenal: to attempt to list these would occupy years of research, and would be perpetually incomplete, with recurring addenda to its many volumes.

For a single drug used in 1950, for any illness for example hypertension, there are, in 1994, dozens, with perhaps ten trade names for each.

In Trinidad and Tobago, we have witnessed the disappearance of smallpox and of endemic malaria, and the almost complete suppression of tuberculosis, leprosy, typhoid and hookworm which were important scourges when I was a boy, and were prevalent when I started practice in 1950. Yet, infestations, like scabies, have increased tremendously and severe acute respiratory ailments continue to incapacitate. Thanks to the availability of antibiotics – increased from four in 1950 to many hundreds in 1994 – these are seldom fatal.

There has been a dramatic increase in diabetes, hypertension and coronary disease. There has been a coincident exacerbation of psychological stress among our population. So-called 'modernisation' and an accelerated lifestyle are taking their toll. Sexual promiscuity and AIDS abound *in tandem*.

Our basic infrastructure has not kept pace with our expanding fundamental needs, for example: flood damage to crops, livestock and property (but providentially not directly to human life), is greater now than at the middle of the century, and, paradoxically, water, both potable and for common use, is scarcer than fifty years ago.

My medical *alma mater*, the San Fernando Hospital and the Port of Spain Institution, continue to suffer from chronic debility and perpetual exhaustion. Doctors are still leaving because of dissatisfaction with conditions.

Our public health is at the mercy of our lop-sided economic development which in turn is dictated by our ineffective and unrepresentative[18], pseudo-democratic, political arrangements.

Public sentiment and the media provide escapism from the realities of survival, by the magnification of superficialities: the sound and fury of steel band vs harmonium in schools which close for weeks because of lack of water or toilets. Months of media discussion regarding the wearing of the 'hijab' in competition with the school uniform succeed in blanketing all consideration of escalating violent crime and cocaine.

In our microcosm, all the ills, frustrations and demands, of all the continents, countries and cultures of our planet Earth are focused in sharp detail.

Prices of foodstuffs and medicines have escalated, often beyond the reach of more than half of our people.

In the midst of all this, I must guiltily confess that for me, personally, life has been very pleasant during the past decade.

While in my political endeavours I have had a share of arrest, victimisation and incarceration, my medical practice has always been full of interest, satisfaction and gratification.

I am now free to pursue all my delights in the evening and at nights, without disturbance – no midnight knocking at my door by patients or police. I leave for the office, twelve miles away, at 8 a.m., and make it, at a leisurely pace, in thirty-five minutes. I close up shop promptly at 3 p.m., unless an emergency arrives at that time. There are eight doctors in Siparia alone, and the daily work load is light. My income pays all my meagre expenses, I have no debts or mortgages to pay, but at my age I resent having to pay income tax. Surely, very senior citizens who have no government pension should be exempt!

From my roof-top patio – my oasis in the arid economic and socio-political desert – I have a lovely 360-degree panoramic view: on the North, the Gulf of Paria, Pointe-a-Pierre, Point Lisas, the City of San Fernando, the Central Range and, beyond all that, the glorious Northern Range, with El Tucuche towering on the horizon.

---

[18] Governments have consistently rejected a proportional representation system for our Parliament, so that sections of our population continue to be un- or under represented.

Oh, how I wish that our talented and beautiful people would more fully appreciate all the natural attributes and bountiful resources of our country, and develop them for the welfare of future generations.

I have a little orchard of mangoes, coconuts, citrus and a sapodilla tree. I also have a charming and cooperative spouse.

And so, I contentedly, with a curious mixture of hope and trepidation, await the twenty-first century and its uncertain future.